70 Years of Levothyroxine

George J. Kahaly

Editor

70 Years of Levothyroxine

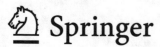 Springer

Editor
George J. Kahaly
Department of Medicine I
Johannes Gutenberg University (JGU) Medical Center
Mainz, Rheinland-Pfalz
Germany

This book is an open access publication.
ISBN 978-3-030-63279-3   ISBN 978-3-030-63277-9   (eBook)
https://doi.org/10.1007/978-3-030-63277-9

This Springer imprint is published by the registered company Springer Nature Switzerland AG
The registered company address is: Gewerbestrasse 11, 6330 Cham, Switzerland

Preface

Levothyroxine (LT4) is celebrating its 70th birthday, since its introduction to the management of hypothyroidism or primary thyroid failure.

This is a good opportunity to explore the history and the current state of the art with regard to the therapeutic use of LT4, now one of the most-prescribed treatments worldwide. In our book, we explore the early research that led to an understanding of the role of thyroid gland that led to the initial therapeutic use of LT4. We also describe the pharmacokinetics, pharmacodynamics and mechanism of action of LT4, its actions on key target organs (heart and bone), and its use and effects in important special populations (children, older persons, pregnancy, and survivors of thyroid cancer). A concluding chapter summarizes pragmatic recommendations for the practicing physician on the optimal clinical application of LT4 substitution.

As the Editor of this book, I am extremely grateful to the nine internationally respected physicians and clinical researchers in the field of thyroid research, based in three continents (Asia, Europe, and the Americas), who agreed to join me to make up our expert Faculty. They were Drs. Takashi Akamizu (Japan), Tomasz Bednarczuk (Poland), Bernadette Biondi (Italy), Gabriela Brenta (Argentina), James Hennessey (USA), Hans-Peter Lipp (Germany), Kris Poppe (Belgium), Salman Razvi (United Kingdom), and Weiping Teng (China). Their expertise, knowledge, and active participation greatly facilitated my task as book Editor. Their important contributions, well-taken points, constructive comments, and excellent proposals made this book possible. This book also benefited from independent peer review by two experts in the field of thyroidology, in addition to the experience and knowledge of our faculty.

I also thank our medical writer, Dr. Mike Gwilt. Mike provided effective editorial support to our Faculty, from the building of the first draft through successive revisions, to the final book you see here. His engagement with the authors—including myself—helped greatly in bringing their knowledge and experience to the page. His engagement with me as Editor helped me to oversee the production of a book of ten coherent chapters that not only stand individually as expert reviews in our authors' fields of expertise, but also work together tell us the full story of seven decades of therapeutic use of LT4.

The idea for this anniversary book, and logistical support, came from Merck Healthcare KGaA, Darmstadt, Germany. I am most grateful to Dr. Bogumila Urgatz (Medical Director) and Dr. Ulrike Hostalek (Executive Medical Director, GMA, GM & Endocrinology) from this company, for this productive and successful collaboration.

Enjoy the reading!

With all best wishes,

Mainz, Rheinland-Pfalz, Germany   George J. Kahaly

Contents

About the Editor and Contributors

Editor

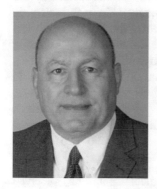

George J. Kahaly, MD, PhD Professor of Medicine and Endocrinology/Metabolism and Director of the Molecular Thyroid Research Laboratory, at the Johannes Gutenberg University (JGU) Medical Center, Mainz, Germany. Dr. Kahaly directs the endocrine and thyroid autoimmunity program at the JGU endocrine outpatient clinic and chairs the ORPHAN referral expert center for Graves' orbitopathy and autoimmune polyendocrinopathy.

He has authored 281 original papers and reviews, covering clinical, experimental, and immune genetic aspects of endocrine autoimmunity, as well as cardiovascular involvement of metabolic disorders, in leading journals, including the *New England Journal of Medicine, The Lancet, JAMA, Annals of Internal Medicine, Clinical Chemistry,* the *Journal of Autoimmunity,* the *Journal of Clinical Endocrinology and Metabolism (JCEM),* the *Journal of Nuclear Medicine, Endocrinology, Thyroid, Endocrine Reviews, Nature Reviews,* and *Autoimmunity Reviews* (current citation H index 48, 8768 citations).

Dr. Kahaly is the 2019 recipient of the American Association of Clinical Endocrinologists/American College of Endocrinology (AACE/ACE) Endocrinology Award and is the 2019 recipient of the British Thyroid Association "George Murray Award" medal. Further awards: include Research Program of the German Endocrine Society (2006, 2008); Poster prize, German

Society of Internal Medicine (2006, 2008); Poster prize, German Endocrine Society (2009); Investigator Award of the European Thyroid Association (2009); Investigator Award of the German Ophthalmic Society (2011); Best Reviewer Award, *European Thyroid Journal* (2018); and British Medical Association Medical Book Award (2018).

Dr. Kahaly is Treasurer and Principal Officer of the European Group on Graves' orbitopathy, and a member of the Editorial Board of the European Thyroid Journal, and the Publication Core Committee of the American Endocrine Society (2020–2023). Other recent posts include Editor of the *Journal of Clinical Endocrinology and Metabolism* (2015–2019), Associate Editor of *Thyroid* (2009–2012), Treasurer and Principal Officer of the Executive Committee of the European Thyroid Association (2007–2016), membership of the scientific program organizing committees of the 2020 International Thyroid Congress, Xian, China, and the 2020 spring meeting of the American Thyroid Association (ATA), and the Executive Committee of the German Thyroid Board (2005–2011), as well as numerous ATA Committees (Laboratory Services Committee [2018–2022], Public Health [2015–2018], Research [2012–2015], Finance and Audit [2007–2011], and Membership and Publication Committees [2000–2006]).

Disclosures: The JGU Medical Center has received research-associated funding from, and GJK consults for, Merck Healthcare KGaA.

Department of Medicine I, Johannes Gutenberg University (JGU) Medical Center, Mainz, Rheinland-Pfalz, Germany

Contributors

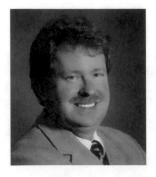

Hans-Peter Lipp, PharmD, PhD Professor for Pharmacoeconomics and Pharmacoepidemiology at the Pharmaceutical Institute of the University of Tübingen. There, I participate in the education of students as a teaching practitioner, with a focus on judgment analyses for accurate selection of therapies.

My research has focused on the clinical pharmacokinetic behavior (including drug–drug interactions) of a broad spectrum of available drugs, based on more than 200 publications in diverse fields, including hemostasis, hemato-oncology, mycology, ophthalmology, endocrinology, and many others. As a director of a large hospital pharmacy within the University Clinic of Tübingen, Germany, I am co-responsible for the dynamic revision of the established drug formulary, especially when drugs and formulations are added, switched, or removed. I am also responsible for continuous negotiations of purchasing conditions, which are very associated closely with the drugs' pharmacology and quality, especially for novel therapeutics.

Disclosures: Professor Lipp has no relationships with or financial interests in any commercial companies related to this book.

University Hospital Tübingen, Tübingen, Germany

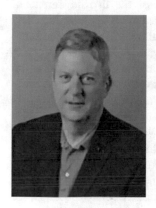

James V. Hennessey, MD Director of Clinical Endocrinology at Beth Israel Deaconess Medical Center and Associate Professor of Medicine at the Harvard Medical School. He graduated from the Medical Faculty of the Karl Franzens University of Graz, Austria. He completed a Medical Residency at the New Britain Hospital in Connecticut. He served with the US Air Force (USAF) as an Internist/Flight Surgeon and later subspecialty training in endocrinology and metabolism at the Walter Reed Army Medical Center in Washington, DC, where he conducted research in thyroxine bioequivalence.

Dr. Hennessey served as the Chief of Endocrinology at USAF Medical Center Wright-Patterson in Ohio and later joined the faculty at Wright State University School of Medicine as the Director of Clinical Clerkships, maintaining a clinical-teaching practice at Wright State and in thyroidology at Wright-Patterson Medical Center. Upon arrival at Brown Medical School in Providence, RI, he transferred to the Air National Guard as a flight surgeon and finally as Rhode Island State Surgeon, retiring after a 25-year USAF career in 2006. While at Brown, he was Associate Director for Clinical Education in the Division of Endocrinology at Rhode Island Hospital and directed the Medical School Endocrine Pathophysiology course.

His career has focused on the clinical education of medical students, resident physicians in internal medicine, and fellows in endocrinology and metabolism. In this capacity, he has conducted lectures, precepted clinical care, and carried out original and sponsored clinical research with his trainees. Currently, he is pursuing his clinical interest in thyroid disease and osteoporosis with both expanding clinical programs.

Disclosures: Dr. Hennessey has consulted for AbbVie, Allergan, and Spetrix for clinical trial design and as an invited speaker on bioequivalence for Merck Healthcare KGaA.

Harvard Medical School, Division of Endocrinology, Beth Israel Deaconess Medical Center, **Boston, MA, USA**

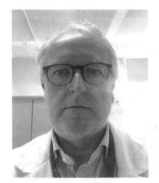

Kris Gustave Poppe, MD, PhD Head of the endocrine unit and coordinator of the thyroid outpatient clinic and research unit at the University Hospital CHU St-Pierre, a teaching hospital from the Université Libre de Bruxelles (ULB), in downtown Brussels.

For more than 20 years, my research is focused on the relationship between thyroid disorders and pregnancy, in particular on the impact of thyroid disorders on female infertility and subsequent treatment with assisted reproductive technology.

I have published more than 70 original and review papers, gave plenary lectures at many European Thyroid and Endocrine meetings, and "meet the Professor" sessions at Endocrine Society meetings. In addition, I have served as a member of the Executive Board of the European Thyroid Association (2008–2012) and coordinator of the Belgian Thyroid Club (2009–2015), and currently serve as a member of the Editorial Board of the European Thyroid Journal.

Disclosures: I received lecture fees from the IBSA Institut Biochimique SA (satellite meeting of the European Thyroid Association) in 2016 and the Berlin-Chemie AG company (ETA educational thyroid meeting) in 2017–2018 and 2020. I have no direct conflict of interest in relation to this book.

Endocrine Unit, Centre Hospitalier Universitaire Saint Pierre, Brussels, Belgium

Université Libre de Bruxelles (ULB), Brussels, Belgium

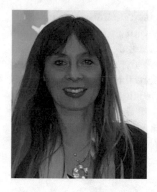

Gabriela Brenta, MD, PhD Staff member of the Department of Endocrinology and Metabolism at Dr. Cesar Milstein Care Unit in Buenos Aires, where she coordinates the Thyroid Unit and holds the rank of Assistant Professor at the Medical School of the University of Buenos Aires. Her areas of interest in clinical research include the cardiovascular and metabolic effects of thyroid hormones, the field of thyroid nodular disease and, in particular, the study of thyroid diseases in the elderly. Original papers and reviews have been published in peer-reviewed journals, including *Thyroid, Endocrine, Nature* and the *Journal of Clinical Endocrinology and Metabolism*. She is a member of the Argentine Society of Endocrinology and Metabolism (SAEM) with an active participation at its Thyroid Department.

She is also member of the editorial board of the peer-reviewed journals, Thyroid and Journal of Endocrinology Investigation. In June 2019, Dr. Brenta completed her term as President of the Latin American Thyroid Society (LATS) and is now engaged on behalf of LATS in the Scientific Committee of the 16th International Thyroid Congress and also in the 19th International Congress of Endocrinology.

Disclosures: Professor Brenta declared no conflict of interest with regard to this book.

Dr. Cesar Milstein Hospital, Buenos Aires, Argentina

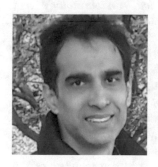

Salman Razvi, MD, FRCP Senior Lecturer in Endocrinology at Newcastle University and a Consultant Endocrinologist at Queen Elizabeth Hospital. He completed his higher medical degrees and specialist training in the North East of England. His doctoral thesis was based on assessing cardiovascular risk in subclinical hypothyroidism. Subsequent to this, he has continued to pursue research evaluating the action of thyroid hormones particularly on the cardiovascular system. The focus of his research has been on investigating the association of thyroid function with cardiovascular events in various populations.

He is the chief investigator of several projects funded by various statutory funding bodies as well as charities.

His main research programs include investigating treatment of subclinical hypothyroidism with thyroid hormones in acute myocardial infarction and age-appropriate treatment of hypothyroidism in the elderly. He has authored more than 75 peer-reviewed publications, relating mainly to thyroid dysfunction.

Dr. Razvi is a member of the editorial board of *Thyroid, Frontiers in Endocrinology* and the *Journal of Endocrinological Investigations*. He is also the Director of Research and Development at Gateshead Hospitals and the Speciality Group Lead for Metabolic and Endocrine Research at the North East and North Cumbria Local Clinical Research Network.

Disclosures: Dr. Razvi has received speaker fees from Merck Healthcare KGaA, Abbott India Pharmaceuticals (Pvt) Ltd., and Berlin-Chemie Ltd., manufacturers of levothyroxine.

Translational and Clinical Research Institute, University of Newcastle, Newcastle-upon-Tyne, UK

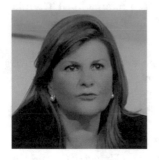

Bernadette Biondi, MD Full professor of internal medicine at the University of Naples "Federico II," where she researches cardiovascular endocrinology and clinical thyroidology, with a special focus on subclinical thyroid dysfunction.

Professor Biondi is author and co-author of numerous papers in leading peer-reviewed journals, including the *Journal of Clinical Endocrinology and Metabolism, European Journal of Endocrinology, Annals of Internal Medicine, Circulation, Nature Clinical Practice in Endocrinology and Metabolism*, the *New England Journal of Medicine, Endocrine Reviews, JAMA, The Lancet*, and the *Journal of the American College of Cardiology*. She also authors the chapter "Endocrine Disorders and Cardiovascular Disease" in the book, *Braunwald's Heart Disease*.

Professor Biondi serves as Associate Editor of *Clinical Thyroidology*. She is also a member of the Awards Committee Roster of the American Thyroid Association and chaired the task force of the European Thyroid Association for the development of clinical practice guidelines on the diagnosis and treatment of subclinical hyperthyroidism.

Disclosures: This research was not supported by external funding and did not receive any specific grant from any funding agency in the public, commercial, or not-for-profit sector.

Professor of Endocrinology and Internal Medicine, University of Naples Federico II, Naples, Italy

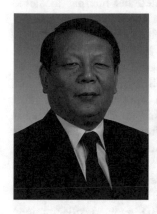

Weiping Teng, MD Professor of Medicine at The First Hospital of China Medical University, Shenyang, and also the Chief of the Institute of Endocrinology of China Medical University and the Chief of State Key Laboratory (Cultivation Base) for Endocrine diseases. Dr. Teng was graduated from China Medical University in 1976. He completed his postdoctoral fellowship training in endocrinology at the University of Cambridge, UK (1988–1990) and at the University of Toronto, Canada (1994–1995).

His key research orientation is thyroid diseases, especially in the fields of epidemiology, the relationship between iodine excess and thyroid diseases, genetics of Graves' disease, autoimmune thyroid diseases, the relationship between pregnancy and thyroid diseases, and the effects of thyroid hormone on brain development. He has published more than 300 articles including in peer-reviewed journals. He considers that the article, "Effect of iodine intake on thyroid diseases in China," published in the *New England Journal of Medicine* (doi: https://doi.org/10.1056/NEJMoa054022) is especially representative of his work.

Currently, Dr. Teng is the Predecessor President of Chinese Endocrine Society (CES). He is also Vice President of AOTA (Asia and Oceania Thyroid Association), the member of ATA (American Thyroid Association) and TES (The Endocrine Society), and the member of editorial board of Thyroid.

Disclosures: Dr. Teng declared no conflict of interest with regard to this book.

First Hospital of China Medical University, Shenyang, China

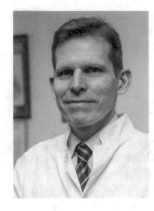

Tomasz Bednarczuk, MD, PhD Professor of Medicine and head of the Department of Internal Medicine and Endocrinology at the Medical University of Warsaw. The department is one of the referral centers in Poland for treatment of patients with various endocrine disorders, including thyroid, parathyroid, adrenal and neuroendocrine tumors.

Dr. Bednarczuk completed his internal medicine and endocrinology training in Warsaw and spent 3 years at the Thyroid Eye Disease Laboratory, Allegheny-Singer Research Institute, Pittsburgh, USA (supervisor Prof. Jack Wall) and Division of Endocrinology and Metabolism, University School of Medicine, Kurume, Japan (supervisor Prof. Yuji Hiromatsu). He received his Ph.D. in 1998 and his habilitation degree in 2004 from the Medical Research Center, Polish Academy of Science.

Dr. Bednarczuk is a clinical scientist with a special research focus on the pathogenesis of Graves' orbitopathy and the genetics of Graves' disease (GD). His research on the genetics of GD involved collaborations with various centers in Europe and Japan. He has published more than 100 papers in peer-reviewed journals.

Dr. Bednarczuk serves as Treasurer of the European Thyroid Association. Moreover, he is a member of the executive committees of the Polish Society of Endocrinology and the Polish Thyroid Association.

Disclosures: Dr. Bednarczuk declared no conflict of interest with regard to this book.

Department of Internal Diseases and Endocrinology, Medical University of Warsaw, Warsaw, Poland

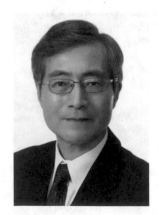

Takashi Akamizu, MD, PhD Professor Emeritus of Wakayama Medical University and Vice President of Kuma Hospital. He obtained his MD and PhD from Kyoto University School of Medicine and completed 3-year postgraduate training at the National Institute of Diabetes and Digestive and Kidney Disorders at the US National Institutes of Health.

He is currently the President of Japan Endocrine Society (JES), the President of Asia-Oceania Thyroid Association (AOTA), and the former President of Japan Thyroid Association (JTA). He received several awards from all these associations including the JES Award of the Japan Endocrine Society, Nagataki-Fujifilm Prize of AOTA and Shichijo/Miyake Awards (JTA), etc. He is an Associate Editor of JCEM and an Editorial member of the Thyroid. His major research interests include pathogenesis and pathophysiology of autoimmune thyroid disease, management of thyroid storm, translational research on ghrelin and IgG4-related disease.

Disclosures: Professor Akamizu declared no conflict of interest with regard to this book.

Wakayama Medical University, Wakayama, Japan

Kuma Hospital, Kobe, Japan

Therapeutic Use of Levothyroxine: A Historical Perspective

George J. Kahaly

The therapeutic use of levothyroxine (LT4) arose from observations made in the second half of the nineteenth century that linked the severe physical and cognitive defects of cretinism with an under-developed, or absent, thyroid gland. Improved outcomes for these subjects following empirical treatment with crude thyroid extracts spurred further research, and isolation, characterisation, and chemical synthesis of LT4 and triiodothyronine (T3) followed in the first half of the twentieth century. Treatment with LT4 + T3 combinations superseded the use of thyroid extracts from the 1960s onwards. The development of reliable and specific assays for thyroid hormones contributed greatly to understanding the importance and function of the thyroid and facilitated individualised treatment. Monotherapy with LT4 has been the mainstay of management of hypothyroidism from about 1970. Thyroid research is far from complete, however, and further research into several outstanding clinical issues will continue to shape LT4-based therapy in the future.

1 Introduction

In the opening chapter of this book, we consider the history of the therapeutic use of levothyroxine (LT4). Recognition of the therapeutic value of LT4 emerged from experience gained from, essentially, empirical administration by physicians of crude thyroid extracts to people with advanced sequelae of hypothyroidism [1–4]. These clinical experiments arose from early studies of people we would today describe as having severe congenital hypothyroidism. Accordingly, our story begins in the

G. J. Kahaly (✉)
Department of Medicine I, Johannes Gutenberg University (JGU) Medical Center,
Mainz, Rheinland-Pfalz, Germany
e-mail: gkahaly@uni-mainz.de

© The Author(s) 2021
G. J. Kahaly (ed.), *70 Years of Levothyroxine*,
https://doi.org/10.1007/978-3-030-63277-9_1

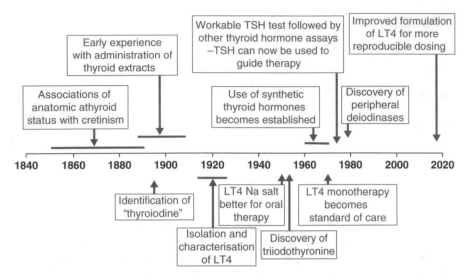

Fig. 1 Overview of key events relevant to the history of therapeutic use of levothyroxine for hypothyroidism. *LT4* levothyroxine, *Na* sodium. Times are approximate

latter half of the nineteenth century, when these pioneering observations were being made, continues to the current management of hypothyroidism with LT4 and concludes with a brief review of outstanding research issues in this fast-moving field. Fig. 1 provides a timeline of key events along this journey, and these important advances are described below.

2 Early Beginnings: Growing Understanding of the Thyroid

2.1 Cretinism, Goitre, and the Recognition of the Importance of the Thyroid Gland

An appreciation of thyroid disease as a clinical entity began during the second half of the nineteenth century [1–4]. Briefly, sporadic, and widely spaced, reports in medical journals during this period described young, short-lived individuals presenting with growth retardation and "sporadic cretinism", which were found to be associated with minimal or absent thyroid tissue [5–7]. Such cases today would be described as congenital hypothyroidism, with the term "sporadic" used to differentiate them from "endemic cretinism", associated with goitre in iodine-deficient regions, which had been described centuries before. Later work during this period introduced the term, "myxoedema", to describe the anatomic appearance of the thyroid in these patients [1].

Surgery to remove goitre was being performed at this time, for example, to relieve symptoms of compression in the neck, despite a continuing lack of understanding of the function of the thyroid gland [8]. One contemporary study showed that removal of the entire thyroid led to the development of symptoms resembling those of "sporadic cretinism", and this observation led the author to restrict future surgeries to partial resection of the thyroid, with better outcomes [9]. Elsewhere, thyroidectomy in animals was shown to produce symptoms reminiscent of myxoedema, providing further strength to the association of athyroid status with "sporadic cretinism" [10]. These extreme cases were the first demonstrations of the pathophysiological importance of the thyroid gland to healthy development although not based on any understanding of the function of the thyroid. Other experiments conducted at this time noted that thyroidectomy was lethal to dogs, but that the health of the animals could be preserved temporarily by grafting the thyroid elsewhere in the animals' bodies [11]. Even so, it was assumed that the function of the thyroid was allied to detoxification of the blood, rather than to an independent and specific endocrine function [3].

2.2 An Endocrine Function for the Thyroid Gland

It had been suggested in about 1820 (soon after the characterisation of iodine as a chemical element) that the limited efficacy of dietary ingestion of foodstuffs such as sponges or seaweed in the diet (an ancient, traditional remedy for goitre) was connected to the presence of iodine in these items [12]. The first attempts at iodine supplementation, either using a tincture of iodine, or with iodised salt, followed during the following decade [4]. A correlation between scarcity of iodine in the environment and an increased prevalence of goitre was published some 30 years later [13]. This was followed by further trials of iodine supplementation in three Departments of France where problems with goitre were especially severe. These were largely successful, and it was reported in 1869 that about 80% of cases of goitre responded favourably to treatment [14]. Several problems with the conduct of these trials led to their early cessation; these included an excessively high dose of iodine (which commonly caused hyperthyroidism in adult recipients), continuing scepticism among the medical profession, and reluctance to participate by citizens who feared that curing their sons' goitres would remove an obstacle to their being conscripted for military service [4].

From about 1890 onwards, physicians were experimenting with the administration of thyroid extracts (orally or subcutaneously) to people with myxoedema [3]. These early clinical studies were generally successful; one patient with advanced myxoedema that developed in middle age was treated with subcutaneous injections of sheep thyroid extract and lived for 28 years before dying of heart failure at age 74 years [15]. The author, the British physician, George Murray, concluded that the thyroid is "purely an internal secretory gland", that the "functions of this gland in man can be fully and permanently carried on by the continued supply of thyroidal hormones", and, crucially, that "duration of life need not be shortened by atrophy of the thyroid gland provided this substitution treatment is fully maintained" [15]. These concepts underpin the management of hypothyroidism to this day. Interestingly, this represents an early example of the seeking of informed consent for a trial of a therapeutic agent: the physician had explained the experimental nature of the treatment and had sought and obtained the patient's consent. A review of 100 cases of patients with myxoedema and cretinism, published in 1893 attests to

Fig. 2 Chemical structures of thyroid hormones

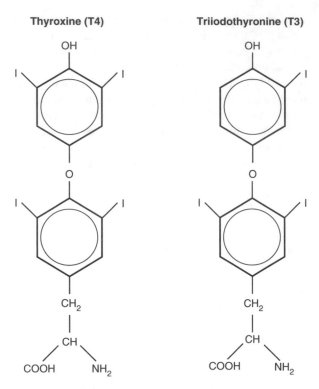

the remarkable success attributed to this treatment, using phrases such as "*complete transformation*" and "*the patient has ceased to be a patient*" [16].

The discovery in 1895 of a substance containing high concentrations of iodine within the thyroid gland ("thyroiodine") was therefore of considerable interest in unifying concepts relating to hypothyroidism and iodine, and the role of the thyroid as an endocrine organ [17]. The substance that would come to be known as thyroxine (T4) was isolated in the USA in 1915 and fully chemically characterised in 1926 (and published the following year [18]). It was also established that LT4 had greater biological activity than a racemic mixture. The discovery of triiodothyronine (T3) as a "normal constituent of the organic iodine fraction of the plasma" of subjects with normal thyroid function or hyperthyroidism followed in 1952 [19]. Fig. 2 shows the chemical structures of these hormones.

3 Towards the Modern Era in the Management of Hypothyroidism

3.1 Introduction of Chemically Synthesised Thyroid Hormones

The early attempts at thyroid replacement via "organ therapy" (as the practice of administration of extracts of animal organs became known), described briefly in the previous section, were taking place at a time when this practice was becoming widespread in the management of other conditions [20]. For example, a report by a leading physician in France on the allegedly rejuvenating effects of self-injection with animal testicular extracts led to great enthusiasm for this practice among other physicians. Eventually, a growing association with widespread quackery in the hands of other practitioners led to a general discrediting of the principle of "organo-therapy" [20, 21].

Nevertheless, although early practitioners such as Murray switched from injected to oral preparations of thyroid extracts, mainly to prevent serious systemic adverse reactions and abscesses and other problems at the local injection site, it was some time before chemically synthesised LT4 entered into clinical practice. This was partly due to limitations of chemically synthesised LT4, which was produced as an acid and had limited bioavailability before the synthesis of a sodium salt of in 1949 [21]. This preparation entered clinical use in that year in the USA, and entered clinical use in Europe some years later.

It took considerable time for synthesised LT4 to become the mainstay of treatment for hypothyroidism, however. Indeed, the use of products based on thyroid extracts did not decline markedly until the latter part of the 1960s, due to difficulties with reproducibility of their biological action and limited storage life [2, 22]. Desiccated thyroid products are available for therapeutic use to this day, despite the currently high regulatory standards for manufacture of LT4 tablets, which ensure reproducibility of day-to-day dosing (see below). Such preparations have persisted, despite lack of convincing objective evidence of superior efficacy in controlling hypothyroid symptoms [23]. There is an enduring perception that these products are a more "natural" treatment than the pharmaceutical preparation [24] although the balance of T4 and T3 levels in animals is not the same as that in humans, and preparations contain excipients and other non-natural substances, as does any pharmaceutical [22].

3.2 Monotherapy or Combination Therapy?

In the 1960s, the use of oral combinations of LT4 and T3 became widely used in the management of hypothyroidism, due to an assumption that delivery of both thyroid hormones would mimic the natural function of the thyroid gland [25]. In addition, as thyroid extracts were essentially the reference product for clinical trials at this time, studies comparing thyroid extracts and LT4 + combinations gave broadly similar clinical results. However, the pharmacokinetic half-life of T3 is much shorter than that of T4 [26]. In addition, it was discovered in the 1970s that about 80% of T3 in peripheral tissues is derived from local conversion from T4 by local deiodinases, rather than from the thyroid [27]. Moreover, too high a dose of T3 results in symptoms of hyperthyroidism, complicating the delivery of combination therapy [26]. A series of clinical trials from 1970 onwards compared T4 + T3 combination therapy with monotherapy with LT4 in hypothyroid patients, and these studies have established monotherapy with LT4 as the standard of care for managing hypothyroidism for the vast majority of patients [28, 29]. Today, LT4 is the most commonly prescribed medication in the USA [30]. A fuller account of the current status of and prospects for LT4 + T3 combination therapy is given in the chapter, "Pharmacodynamic and Therapeutic Actions of Levothyroxine" of this book.

3.3   Technological Advances: Better Assays of Thyroid Function

The introduction of pharmaceutical preparations of synthetic thyroid hormones and establishment of monotherapy with LT4 as the standard of care for hypothyroidism opened up a prospect of delivery of stable, reproducible therapy tailored to the needs of the individual patient. To achieve this, it was necessary to measure circulating levels of thyroid hormones accurately and reproducibly. In the 1950s, the only thyroid hormone test available (the protein bound iodine assay) provided an indirect measurement of serum total T4; today, sensitive and specific assays exist for free and bound T4 or T3, thyrotropin (thyroid-stimulating hormone; TSH), thyroglobulin (a precursor of thyroid hormones), and a range of proteins that bind thyroid hormones in the circulation, based on radioimmunoassay or liquid chromatography-tandem mass spectrometry (LC-MS/MS) technology [31]. These assays made it possible to accurately determine the thyroid status of patients with all degrees of severity of thyroid dysfunction and facilitated a leap in our understanding of the physiology of the thyroid gland.

The discovery of a workable TSH test in the mid 1970s was a key development in the diagnosis and management of hypothyroidism. Levels of T4 and T3 are low in the setting of hypothyroidism, and the pituitary responds by increasing the secretion of TSH in an attempt to correct this, leading to an abnormally high TSH level [25]. The relationship between levels of T4 and TSH is not linear, however, as decreasing the level of T4 by half results in an increase in the TSH level of as much as 100-fold [32]. Large changes in TSH are clearly more amenable to accurate measurement than the accompanying relatively much smaller changes in T4. Accordingly, the management of hypothyroidism is now based on normalisation of the circulating TSH level to within a reference range for this parameter derived from a healthy population [33–35].

3.4   Recent Developments in Levothyroxine Therapy

LT4 was introduced into the therapeutic armamentarium in the USA in the 1950s without a requirement for regulatory oversight. This situation is very different today, with increasingly close regulatory attention paid to the standards of manufacture of LT4 products. This has led to the development of new formulations of LT4, with more accurate and reproducible dosing, designed to improve the accuracy and reproducibility of exposure to LT4 for a patient taking this medication. A full account of this new formulation is given in the following chapter [36].

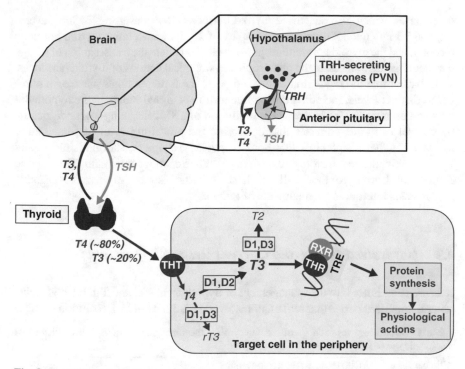

Fig. 3 Simplified schematic overview of the principal physiological systems involved in thyroid hormone homeostasis. *D1/2/3* deiodinase 1/2/3, *T2* diiodothyronine, *rT3* reverse triiodothyronine (inactive), *RXR* retinoic acid receptor, *TRE* thyroid hormone response element, *T3* triiodothyronine, *T4* thyroxine, *THR* thyroid hormone receptor, *TRH* thyrotropin-releasing hormone, *TSH* thyrotropin (thyroid-stimulating hormone), *PVN* periventricular nucleus (of the hypothalamus)

4 Where We Stand Today

4.1 A Fuller (But Incomplete) Understanding of Thyroid Hormone Homeostasis

Our understanding of the complex homeostatic mechanisms underlying the regulation of thyroid hormones and their actions continues to increase. Fig. 3 provides an overview of the principal systems involved [37–40]. Briefly, inputs from physiological processes all around the body are integrated within the hypothalamus. Neurones within the periventricular nucleus of the hypothalamus secrete higher or lower amounts of thyrotropin-releasing hormone (TRH), depending on current physiological needs, which acts on the nearby anterior pituitary gland to promote secretion of TSH, the principal regulator of thyroid hormone secretion. Most (about 80%) of the thyroid hormone secreted by the thyroid in response to TSH is T4, with T3 making up the remainder. T3 and T4 feedback to the hypothalamus and pituitary to inhibit further production of TSH: thus, hypothyroidism is characterised by high levels of TSH, due to lack of inhibition of TSH secretion by thyroid-derived T4.

In the peripheral tissues, thyroid hormone-sensitive target cells of the body take up T4 and T3 via transmembrane carriers. T4 is converted to T3 within cells by specific deiodinases, which also deactivate thyroid hormones, by converting T4 into reverse T3, and T3 into diiodothyronine. A complex of T3, its intracellular thyroid hormone receptor, and the thyroid hormone-responsive element alters the transcription of a large number of genes to mediate the pleiotropic physiological actions of thyroid hormones.

It is clear that the regulation of thyroid hormone function takes place on a number of distinct levels, including during integration of signal inputs in the hypothalamus and secretion of TRH, feedback inhibition of TSH release by T4, and, locally, by control of the deiodinases that determine the prevailing level of functionally active T3. Other chapters of this book, especially chapters, "Administration and Pharmacokinetics of Levothyroxine", and "Pharmacodynamic and Therapeutic Actions of Levothyroxine" will touch on specific aspects of thyroid hormone homeostasis relevant to their subjects of interest.

4.2   Unresolved Issues and Current Research Questions

Research continues into the management of hypothyroidism, and Table 1 highlights several important issues that remain unresolved [28, 32, 41–47]. Resolution of these

Table 1 Outstanding research questions concerning the management of hypothyroidism and therapeutic use of LT4

Clinical issue	Outstanding research questions
Subclinical hypothyroidism	This term describes a mild elevation of TSH where the thyroid-derived hormones are within their normal reference ranges. The current consensus is that most people with subclinical hypothyroidism, and a baseline serum TSH below 10 mU/L, should not receive treatment with LT4 [41]. However, a trial of LT4 may be given to non-elderly patients with symptoms, risk factors for atherosclerosis and coronary heart disease, e.g. hyperlipidaemia, hypertension, diabetes mellitus, and mild elevation of TSH, according to European guidelines [42].
TSH reference ranges	Debate continues as to whether the upper reference limit for serum TSH should be reduced [32].
Cardiovascular disease	People with foremost acute cardiovascular disease have reduced levels of thyroid hormones, particularly T3, on average, and this has been associated with increased risk of adverse clinical outcomes in observational studies [45]. Experts in the field have called for clinical evaluations of thyroid hormone treatment (with LT4 and/or T3) in this population [46]. More data are required on the association between subclinical hypothyroidism and the risk of adverse cardiovascular outcomes [41, 42].
Unwell patients with well-controlled TSH	Some patients report symptoms reminiscent of thyroid dysfunction despite well-controlled thyroid hormones [47]. Many of these symptoms will be found to relate to a non-thyroid cause, and can be eliminated through careful patient workup [47]. However, patients may have their own individual set point for thyroid hormone levels, and the delivery of individualised therapy for this population requires further study [32].
LT4 monotherapy, or LT4 + T3?	Current guidance does not support the use of combinations of LT4 and T3 to correct hypothyroidism (see text). However, some experts support the use of a trial of LT4 + T3 where patients' symptoms have not been controlled by TSH-optimised LT4 monotherapy and cannot be explained by other conditions [28]. Combination therapy with thyroid hormones remains within the research domain, for now.

clinical issues will influence the future management of hypothyroidism, including the therapeutic use of LT4.

5 Conclusions

The history of hypothyroidism and its management spans the golden age of clinical research, from empirical medical and surgical treatments unencumbered by understanding of thyroid physiology in the nineteenth century to individualised, TSH-guided treatment with LT4 today. Along the way, many clinical and experimental studies, enhancements in technology, and improved LT4 preparations have increased greatly our ability to deliver optimal care for hypothyroidism, based on the therapeutic administration of LT4.

References

1. Lindholm J, Laurberg P. Hypothyroidism and thyroid substitution: historical aspects. J Thyroid Res. 2011;2011:809341.
2. McAninch EA, Bianco AC. The history and future of treatment of hypothyroidism. Ann Intern Med. 2016;164:50–6.
3. Ahmed AM, Ahmed NH. History of disorders of thyroid dysfunction. East Mediterr Health J. 2005;11:459–69.
4. Zimmermann MB. Research on iodine deficiency and goiter in the 19th and early 20th centuries. J Nutr. 2008;138:2060–3.
5. Curling TB. Two cases of absence of the thyroid body, and symmetrical swellings of fat tissue at the sides of the neck, connected with defective cerebral development. Med Chir Trans. 1850;33:303–6.
6. Fagge CH. On sporadic cretinism, occurring in England. Med Chir Trans. 1871;54:55–169.
7. Gull WW. On a cretinoid state supervening in adult life in women. Trans Clin Soc Lond. 1874;7:180–5.
8. Hannan SA. The magnificent seven: a history of modern thyroid surgery. Int J Surg. 2006;4:187–91.
9. Kocher T. Ueber Kropf exstirpation und ihre Folgen. Arch Klin Chir. 1883;29:254–335.
10. Horsley V. On the function of the thyroid gland. Proc R Soc Lond. 1885;38:5–7.
11. Schiff M. Résumé d'une nouvelle série d'expériences sur les effets de l'ablation des corps thyroîdes. Rev Med Suisse Romande. 1884;4:425–45.
12. Coindet JF. Nouvelles recherches sur les effets de l'iode et sur les précautions à suivre dans le traitement du goître par ce nouveau remède. Ann Chim Phys. 1821;16(Ser. 2):345–56.
13. Chatin A. Recherches sur l'iode des eaux douces;de la présence de ce corps dans les plantes at les animaux terrestes. C R Hebd Séances Acad Sci. 1851;31:280–3.
14. Goitre in savoy. Lancet. 1869;94:518.
15. Murray GR. The life-history of the first case of myxoedema treated by thyroid extract. Br Med J. 1920;1:359–60.
16. Beadles CF. The treatment of myxoedema and cretinism, being a review of the treatment of these diseases with the thyroid gland, with a table of 100 published cases. J Ment Sci. 1893;39:509–36.

17. Baumann E. Ueber das normale Vorkommen von Jod im Thierkörper. Hoppe-Seyler's Z Physiol Chem. 1895;21:319–30.
18. Harington CR, Barger G. XXIII. Chemistry of thyroxine. III. Constitution and synthesis of thyroxine. Br Med J. 1927;21:169–83.
19. Gross J, Pitt-Rivers R. The identification of 3:5:3′-L-triiodothyronine in human plasma. Lancet. 1952;259:439–41.
20. Bernhardt MS. Organotherapy. JAMA Dermatol. 2013;149:1366.
21. Slater S. The discovery of thyroid replacement therapy. Part 3: a complete transformation. J R Soc Med. 2011;104:100–6.
22. American Thyroid Association. Thyroid hormone treatment. Available at http://www.thyroid.org/thyroid-hormone-treatment/. Accessed Jul 2020.
23. Hoang TD, Olsen CH, Mai VQ, Clyde PW, Shakir MK. Desiccated thyroid extract compared with levothyroxine in the treatment of hypothyroidism: a randomized, double-blind, crossover study. J Clin Endocrinol Metab. 2013;98:1982–90.
24. American Thyroid Association. Clinical thyroidology for patients. Hypothyroidism. Desiccated thyroid extract vs levothyroxine in the treatment of hypothyroidism. Available at https://www.thyroid.org/patient-thyroid-information/ct-for-patients/vol-6-issue-8/vol-6-issue-8-p-3/. Accessed Jul 2020.
25. Kansagra SM, McCudden BSCR, Willis MS. The challenges and complexities of thyroid hormone replacement. Lab Med. 2010;41:338–48.
26. Irizarry I. Thyroid hormone toxicity. Medscape drugs and diseases. Available at https://emedicine.medscape.com/article/819692-overview. Accessed Jul 2020.
27. Luongo C, Dentice M, Salvatore D. Deiodinases and their intricate role in thyroid hormone homeostasis. Nat Rev Endocrinol. 2019;15:479–88.
28. Dayan C, Panicker V. Management of hypothyroidism with combination thyroxine (T4) and triiodothyronine (T3) hormone replacement in clinical practice: a review of suggested guidance. Thyroid Res. 2018;11:1.
29. Wiersinga WM, Duntas L, Fadeyev V, Nygaard B, Vanderpump MP. 2012 ETA guidelines: the use of L-T4 + L-T3 in the treatment of hypothyroidism. Eur Thyroid J. 2012;1:55–71.
30. Frellick M. Top-selling, top-prescribed drugs for 2016. Medscape. 2 Oct 2017. Available at https://www.medscape.com/viewarticle/886404. Accessed Jul 2020.
31. Spencer CA. Assay of thyroid hormones and related substances. Endotext [Internet]. Available at https://www.ncbi.nlm.nih.gov/books/NBK279113/. Accessed Jul 2020.
32. Razvi S, Bhana S, Mrabeti S. Challenges in interpreting thyroid stimulating hormone results in the diagnosis of thyroid dysfunction. J Thyroid Res. 2019;2019:4106816.
33. Okosieme O, Gilbert J, Abraham P, et al. Management of primary hypothyroidism: statement by the British Thyroid Association Executive Committee. Clin Endocrinol (Oxf). 2016;84:799–808.
34. National Institute for Health and Care Excellence. Clinical knowledge summaries. Hypothyroidism. Last revised in Jun 2018. Available at https://cks.nice.org.uk/hypothyroidism. Last accessed Jul 2019.
35. Jonklaas J, Bianco AC, Bauer AJ, et al. Guidelines for the treatment of hypothyroidism: prepared by the American Thyroid Association Task Force on Thyroid Hormone Replacement. Thyroid. 2014;24:1670–751.
36. Lipp HP, Hostalek U. A new formulation of levothyroxine engineered to meet new specification standards. Curr Med Res Opin. 2019;35:147–50.
37. Visser TJ. Cellular uptake of thyroid hormones. Endotext [Internet]. Available at https://www.ncbi.nlm.nih.gov/books/NBK285565/. Accessed Jul 2020.
38. Ortiga-Carvalho TM, Sidhaye AR, Wondisford FE. Thyroid hormone receptors and resistance to thyroid hormone disorders. Nat Rev Endocrinol. 2014;10:582–91.
39. Nillni EA. Regulation of the hypothalamic thyrotropin releasing hormone (TRH) neuron by neuronal and peripheral inputs. Front Neuroendocrinol. 2010;31:134–56.

40. Shahid MA, Ashraf MA, Sharma S. Physiology, thyroid hormone. Stat Pearls [Internet]. 2018. Available at https://www.ncbi.nlm.nih.gov/books/NBK500006/. Accessed Jul 2020.
41. Bekkering GE, Agoritsas T, Lytvyn L, et al. Thyroid hormones treatment for subclinical hypothyroidism: a clinical practice guideline. BMJ. 2019;l2006:365.
42. Pearce SH, Brabant G, Duntas LH, et al. 2013 ETA guideline: management of subclinical hypothyroidism. Eur Thyroid J. 2013;2:215–28.
43. Chaker L, Baumgartner C, den Elzen WP, et al. Thyroid function within the reference range and the risk of stroke: an individual participant data analysis. J Clin Endocrinol Metab. 2016;101:4270–82.
44. Åsvold BO, Vatten LJ, Bjøro T, et al. Thyroid function within the normal range and risk of coronary heart disease: an individual participant data analysis of 14 cohorts. JAMA Intern Med. 2015;175:1037–47.
45. Razvi S, Jabbar A, Pingitore A, et al. Thyroid hormones and cardiovascular function and diseases. J Am Coll Cardiol. 2018;71:1781–96.
46. Razvi S. Novel uses of thyroid hormones in cardiovascular conditions. Endocrine. 2019;66:115–23.
47. Centanni M, Benvenga S, Sachmechi I. Diagnosis and management of treatment-refractory hypothyroidism: an expert consensus report. J Endocrinol Investig. 2017;40:1289–301.

Administration and Pharmacokinetics of Levothyroxine

Hans-Peter Lipp

Lifelong treatment with LT4, guided by levels of thyrotropin, is the mainstay of management of hypothyroidism. The bioavailability of LT4 is about 70% following an oral dose, with absorption occurring mainly in the ileum and jejunum. Maximum plasma concentrations of LT4 are achieved about 3 h after an oral dose in patients with hypothyroidism. The long terminal half-life of orally administered LT4, about 7.5 days, is consistent with once-daily dosing. Pregnancy, several medical conditions (especially) those affecting the gut, and a number of drugs, supplements, or foodstuffs can reduce the absorption and absolute bioavailability of LT4, or can alter the secretion of TSH, with detrimental consequences for long-term control of thyroid function. Poor adherence to LT4 therapy is also a common challenge. The introduction of novel formulations of LT4, with more precise delivery of the active ingredient and higher levels of bioequivalence with existing products will facilitate accurate titration of LT4 for patients with hypothyroidism.

1 Introduction

Oral administration of levothyroxine (LT4), which targets the circulating level of thyrotropin (thyroid-stimulating hormone, TSH) to within a predefined reference range, is the mainstay of treatment of hypothyroidism [1–3]. This chapter summarises the administration, absorption, distribution, metabolism, and elimination of LT4. In addition, it addresses the therapeutic significance of pharmacologic and other factors that can alter exposure to LT4, and of changing regulatory requirements concerning the manufacture of LT4 tablets.

H.-P. Lipp (✉)
University Hospital Tübingen, Tübingen, Germany
e-mail: Hans-Peter.Lipp@med.uni-tuebingen.de

© The Author(s) 2021
G. J. Kahaly (ed.), *70 Years of Levothyroxine*,
https://doi.org/10.1007/978-3-030-63277-9_2

2 Absorption, Distribution, Metabolism, and Elimination of Levothyroxine

2.1 Absorption and Distribution

In general, about 70–80% of an oral dose of LT4 is absorbed from the intestine [4], which may involve transport of the LT4 molecule on the Organic Acid Transporting Polypeptide 2B1 (OATP2B1) transporter [5]. One study did not find significant differences in absorption of LT4 between subjects with and without hypothyroidism, whereas another study demonstrated higher bioavailability of LT4 in subjects with hypothyroidism or hyperthyroidism, compared with euthyroid subjects [6]. It has been shown that about half of an oral dose of the hormone was absorbed in the jejunum and ileum following administration of radiolabelled LT4 [7]. A modest reduction in LT4 absorption was noted in elderly subjects (>70 years), compared with younger adults [8]. In routine clinical practice, titration of the LT4 dose in an elderly patient to an appropriate age-specific reference range would account for this effect of age on LT4 absorption (see chapter, "Levothyroxine in the Older Patient", of this book) [9]. Unlike T4, T3 is essentially completely absorbed (100%) from the intestine following an oral dose [10].

Fig. 1 shows the plasma concentration-time curve from a pharmacokinetic evaluation of two formulations of LT4 in healthy subjects [11]. The time to maximal plasma concentration (T_{max}) of LT4 has been reported as 3 h in subjects with primary

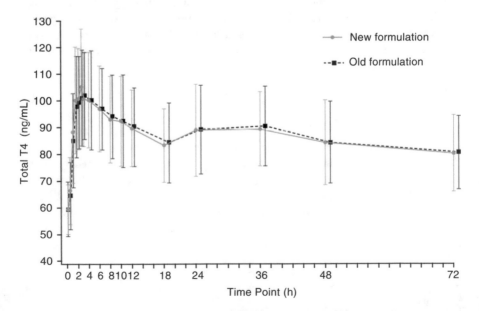

Fig. 1 Plasma concentration-time curves from a comparison of an existing LT4 tablet formulation with a new LT4 tablet formulation designed to meet new regulatory requirements for the manufacture of such products. (Reproduced with permission from Ref. [11])

hypothyroidism and 2 h in euthyroid controls [12]. Concomitant food intake reduces the bioavailability of LT4, hence the labelling requirement to take LT4 tablets on an empty stomach, e.g. 30 min before breakfast, or 3 h after the evening meal [12, 13]. In plasma, LT4 is highly bound to plasma proteins (>99.9%) and distributes within a volume equal approximately to the human body's total extracellular space (about 11–15 L) [14, 15].

2.2 Metabolism and Elimination

The main route of metabolism of LT4, and the route most relevant to its physiological actions, is conversion to T3 and deactivation, mediated by three peripheral deiodinases (Table 1) [16, 17]. Briefly, deiodinases D1 and D2 can mediate the conversion of T4 to T3, enhancing the availability of T3 to local tissues. Accordingly, LT4 may be considered to act largely as a prodrug for delivery of T3 to peripheral tissues. D2 is more important than D1 for generating T3; D1 is especially important for clearing the inactive thyroid hormone metabolite, reverse T3 (rT3), from the system via conversion to a further inactive deiodinated thyroid hormone metabolite. The main function of deiodinase D3 is the degradation of thyroid hormones. Polymorphisms of deiodinases may inhibit the conversion of LT4 to T3 in the periphery and have been proposed to explain an incomplete effect of exogenous LT4 treatment in resolving symptoms of hypothyroidism in some patients [18].

Multiple metabolites of thyroid hormones exist, and some of these may have intriguing biological actions that are the focus of current research [19–21]. Pathways for biotransformation of LT4 include decarboxylation and oxidative deamination, which results in, e.g. 3-iodothyroacetic acid. The biological activity of metabolites of LT4 remains to be established; 3-iodothyroacetic acid, for example, has been shown to induce antidepressant effects, and to promote itching and discomfort, in animal models [21].

Table 1 Metabolism of levothyroxine by peripheral deiodinases

	Deiodinase D1	Deiodinase D2	Deiodinase D3
Mainly expressed in	Liver, kidney, thyroid	Brain, pituitary, skeletal muscle, heart	Widely expressed
Principal reaction	T4 → T3	T4 → T3	T4 → rT3
Other important reactions	T4 → rT3 T3 or rT3 → T2	rT3 → T2	T3 → T2
Summary of physiological importance	• Important source of plasma T3 • Recovery of iodine from inactive thyroid hormone metabolites	• Regulation of local cellular T3 levels • Maintaining pituitary/hypothalamic feedback for thyroid hormone production	• Regulation of local cellular D3 levels, independent of local T3 or T4 levels • Degradation of thyroid hormones

T4 thyroxine, *T3* triiodothyronine, *rT3* reverse triiodothyronine, *T2* 3,3'-diiodothyronine. Compiled from information presented in Refs. [16, 17]

The elimination half-life of LT4 after oral dosing averages 7.5 days in patients with hypothyroidism, consistent with once-daily dosing [14]. A slightly lower elimination half-life was reported in euthyroid subjects (average 6.2 days) [14]. Interestingly, the elimination half-life of T3 is much lower (1–1.4 days, on average) [14], which may complicate future attempts to deliver LT4–T3 combination therapies [22].

3 Factors That May Alter Exposure to an Oral Dose of Levothyroxine

3.1 Factors That May Reduce Exposure to Levothyroxine

3.1.1 Diurnal Variation

Taking LT4 at bedtime (e.g. 3 h after the evening meal) rather than in the morning modestly but significantly increased LT4 levels and reduced TSH levels in the blood [23]. Consequently, it has been proposed to move the routine administration of LT4 from morning to evening, especially as a range of secondary measures (creatinine, lipids, body mass index, heart rate, quality of life) were unchanged between morning and bedtime administration. However, the usually recommended time of intake of LT4 remains in the morning (but at least 30 min before consumption of tea, coffee, or breakfast).

3.1.2 Malabsorption of, and Suboptimal Adherence to, Levothyroxine

Numerous factors may inhibit the absorption of LT4 into the bloodstream, including pre-existing intestinal disorders (e.g. celiac disease, prior gut resection or some forms of bariatric surgery), or concomitant intakes of certain supplements that contain metal ions (e.g. antacids, calcium, iron), drugs (e.g. laxatives, sevelamer, proton pump inhibitors), or soya protein [24–29]. The solubility of LT4 increases as pH decreases [30]. Proton pump inhibitors reduce the acidity (and increase the pH) of the stomach, and thus may reduce the bioavailability of LT4 by about 40% [29]; conversely, co-administration of ascorbic acid (vitamin C) reduces gastric pH and increases the absorption of LT4 [29, 30].

Malabsorption of LT4 results in lower than expected blood levels of LT4 and higher than expected levels of TSH, sometimes even in the setting of high doses of exogenous LT4. Alternative formulations to the usual tablet may be considered for patients with documented LT4 malabsorption [27, 31]. In cases where suboptimal adherence to LT4 therapy is suspected [32], the LT4 absorption test, where thyroid hormone levels are measured after a supervised dose of LT4, can be useful in distinguishing non-adherence of LT4 from genuine cases of malabsorption of LT4 [33].

Intramuscular LT4 treatment has been proposed for patients with severe intestinal malabsorption of LT4 though this approach remains within the research domain at present [34].

3.2 Factors That May Alter the Measured Level of Thyrotropin

A series of other factors influences the TSH test result, and therefore have clinical implications for the administration of LT4. This has been reviewed elsewhere [27], and is summarised briefly as follows:

Pregnancy	The requirement for, and production of, thyroid hormones increase markedly during pregnancy, with a consequent fall in TSH levels. Current guidelines recommend use of locally derived, trimester-specific reference ranges for testing thyroid function in pregnant women [35].
Drugs	Substances that alter the level of TSH will impact on the required dosage of LT4, as the TSH level is used to guide therapy. Several medications have the potential to decrease the TSH result, including dopamine antagonists, glucocorticoids, alemtuzumab, proton pump inhibitors, interferon-alpha, and metformin. Other drugs may increase or decrease the TSH test result, including lithium or amiodarone [27, 36–40].
Biorhythms	TSH secretion follows a diurnal variation, with the lowest value recorded around the middle of the day [41]. A circannual variation in TSH has also been observed in a large database study, with lower values during the summer [42], although the functional significance of this observation remains uncertain [43].
Demographics	TSH levels increase with age and are higher in women vs. men [43, 44]. Ethnicity also influences thyroid hormone levels [43, 44], which adds weight to the importance of using relevant reference populations for determining "normal" TSH results.
Smoking	TSH levels may be lower in smokers vs. non-smokers [45].
Obesity	Obesity is often considered to be a consequence (or a symptom) of hypothyroidism [1]. However, TSH levels correlate positively with BMI, consistent with a mechanism in which increased leptin secretion in obese subjects may drive increased secretion of TSH [46, 47]. The relationships between obesity, the TSH level, and the LT4 requirement are therefore complex.
Interference with TSH assays	Different commercial TSH assays may have different ability to recognise "macro-TSH", which is TSH attached to IgG autoantibodies [48]. Macro-TSH is secreted variably between individuals with hypothyroidism. Other substances in the patient's circulation may interfere directly with the operation of the TSH test, such as autoantibodies to LT4, rheumatoid factors (IgM antibodies directed against human IgG), and heterophilic antibodies (particularly human anti-mouse IgG antibodies [HAMA]), leading to variable test results [49].

4 Levothyroxine Tablets in a Changing Regulatory Environment

The manufacture of pharmaceutical products is subject to regulatory supervision to ensure maintained, high quality and consistency of successive batches; in particular, new formulations of currently available LT4 products must be bioequivalent to the existing formulation [50]. A small change in the level of T4 in the bloodstream will result in a much larger relative change in TSH secretion [28]. Accordingly, LT4 is regarded as a "narrow therapeutic index" drug in Europe (similar terms are used in other countries). According to the standard criteria for bioequivalence between an equivalent oral dose of two pharmaceutical preparations, the 90% confidence intervals (90%CI) for the geometric mean ratio of the area under the concentration-time curve (AUC) and the peak plasma concentration (C_{max}) must be contained between 80% and 125% [51, 52]. For most narrow therapeutic index drugs, including LT4, current specifications now require that the 90% CI for the geometric mean ratio of the AUC and C_{max} values must lie between 90% and 111%, for the products to be considered to be bioequivalent [51, 52]. Updated regulations in several countries now also require the actual LT4 content of LT4 tablets to lie between 90% or 95% (depending on the country) and 105% of the amount declared on the package, throughout the shelf life of the product [53–55].

A randomised clinical trial compared the clinical pharmacokinetics of a new formulation of LT4 that meets these updated, narrowed requirements for bioequivalence with the previous formulation, in 216 healthy subjects [11, 56]. Fig. 1 showed that the plasma concentration-time curves and C_{max} values of the two formulations were essentially identical [11]. A formal evaluation of bioequivalence showed that the new formulation with improved specifications met the updated, stricter criteria for bioequivalence for a new formulation of a narrow therapeutic index drug (Fig. 2).

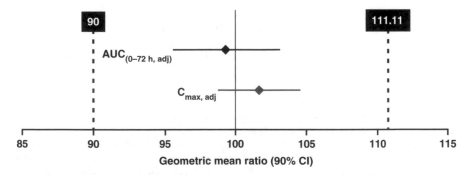

Fig. 2 Formal demonstration of bioequivalence according to updated regulatory criteria between the new and former LT4 tablet formulations shown in Fig. 1. (Reproduced with permission from Ref. [56])

5 Conclusions

LT4 is absorbed well and quickly from the gastrointestinal tract after oral administration. Once-daily dosing is feasible, based on its long half-life. Several medical conditions, particularly those affecting the gut, a number of drugs, pregnancy, and ingestion of supplements or food can interfere with the absorption of LT4 or the corresponding TSH test. As a consequence, care must be taken to identify and exclude these factors, as well as suboptimal adherence to therapy, when a patient presents with symptoms of hypothyroidism in spite of LT4 prescriptions. The introduction of novel formulations of LT4, with improved drug stability over time, more precise delivery of the active ingredient, and higher levels of bioequivalence compared with existing products promises to simplify accurate titration of LT4 for patients with hypothyroidism.

References

1. Okosieme O, Gilbert J, Abraham P, et al. Management of primary hypothyroidism: statement by the British Thyroid Association Executive Committee. Clin Endocrinol (Oxf). 2016;84:799–808.
2. National Institute for Health and Care Excellence. Clinical knowledge summaries. Hypothyroidism. Last revised in June 2018. Available at https://cks.nice.org.uk/hypothyroidism. Last accessed Jul 2019.
3. Jonklaas J, Bianco AC, Bauer AJ, et al. Guidelines for the treatment of hypothyroidism: prepared by the American Thyroid Association Task Force on Thyroid Hormone Replacement. Thyroid. 2014;24:1670–751.
4. Read DG, Hays MT, Hershman JM. Absorption of oral thyroxine in hypothyroid and normal man. J Clin Endocrinol Metab. 1970;30:798–9.
5. Meyer Zu Schwabedissen HE, Ferreira C, Schaefer AM, et al. Thyroid hormones are transport substrates and transcriptional regulators of organic anion transporting polypeptide 2B1. Mol Pharmacol. 2018;94:700–12.
6. Hasselström K, Siersbaek-Nielsen K, Lumholtz IB, Faber J, Kirkegaard C, Friis T. The bioavailability of thyroxine and 3,5,3'-triiodothyronine in normal subjects and in hyper- and hypothyroid patients. Acta Endocrinol (Copenh). 1985;110:483–6.
7. Hays MT. Localization of human thyroxine absorption. Thyroid. 1991;1:241–8.
8. Hays MT, Nielsen KR. Human thyroxine absorption: age effects and methodological analyses. Thyroid. 1994;4:55–64.
9. Leng O, Razvi S. Hypothyroidism in the older population. Thyroid Res. 2019;12:2.
10. Hays MT. Absorption of triiodothyronine in man. J Clin Endocrinol Metab. 1970;30:675–6.
11. Gottwald-Hostalek U, Uhl W, Wolna P, Kahaly GJ. New levothyroxine formulation meeting 95–105% specification over the whole shelf-life: results from two pharmacokinetic trials. Curr Med Res Opin. 2017;33:169–74.
12. Benvenga S, Bartolone L, Squadrito S, Lo Giudice F, Trimarchi F. Delayed intestinal absorption of levothyroxine. Thyroid. 1995;5:249–53.
13. Wenzel KW, Kirschsieper HE. Aspects of the absorption of oral L-thyroxine in normal man. Metabolism. 1977;26:1–8.
14. Nicoloff JT, Low JC, Dussault JH, Fisher DA. Simultaneous measurement of thyroxine and triiodothyronine peripheral turnover kinetics in man. J Clin Invest. 1972;51:473–83.

15. Colucci P, Yue CS, Ducharme M, Benvenga S. A review of the pharmacokinetics of levothyroxine for the treatment of hypothyroidism. Eur Endocrinol. 2013;9:40–7.
16. Peeters RP, Visser TJ. Metabolism of thyroid hormone. Endotext [Internet]. Available at https://www.ncbi.nlm.nih.gov/books/NBK285545. Accessed Jul 2020.
17. Bianco AC, da Conceição RR. The deiodinase trio and thyroid hormone signaling. Methods Mol Biol. 1801;2018:67–83.
18. Bianco AC, Kim BS. Pathophysiological relevance of deiodinase polymorphism. Curr Opin Endocrinol Diabetes Obes. 2018;25:341–6.
19. Köhrle J. The colorful diversity of thyroid hormone metabolites. Eur Thyroid J. 2019;8:115–29.
20. Louzada RA, Carvalho DP. Similarities and differences in the peripheral actions of thyroid hormones and their metabolites. Front Endocrinol (Lausanne). 2018;9:394.
21. Landucci E, Laurino A, Cinci L, Gencarelli M, Raimondi L. Thyroid hormone, thyroid hormone metabolites and mast cells: a less explored issue. Front Cell Neurosci. 2019;13:79.
22. Kansagra SM, McCudden CR, Willis MS. The challenges and complexities of thyroid hormone replacement. Lab Med. 2010;41:338–48.
23. Bolk N, Visser TJ, Nijman J, Jongste IJ, Tijssen JG, Berghout A. Effects of evening vs morning levothyroxine intake: a randomized double-blind crossover trial. Arch Intern Med. 2010;170:1996–2003.
24. Mersebach H, Rasmussen AK, Kirkegaard L, Feldt-Rasmussen U. Intestinal adsorption of levothyroxine by antacids and laxatives: case stories and in vitro experiments. Pharmacol Toxicol. 1999;84:107–9.
25. Sathyapalan T, Manuchehri AM, Thatcher NJ, et al. The effect of soy phytoestrogen supplementation on thyroid status and cardiovascular risk markers in patients with subclinical hypothyroidism: a randomized, double-blind, crossover study. J Clin Endocrinol Metab. 2011;96:1442–9.
26. Fain K, Rojas AP, Peiris AN. Hypothyroidism following gastric sleeve surgery resolved by ingesting crushed thyroxine tablets. Proc (Bayl Univ Med Cent). 2019;33:38–9. eCollection Jan 2020.
27. Castellana M, Castellana C, Giovanella L, Trimboli P. Prevalence of gastrointestinal disorders having an impact on tablet levothyroxine absorption: should this formulation still be considered as the first-line therapy? Endocrine. 2020;67:281–90.
28. Razvi S, Bhana S, Mrabeti S. Challenges in interpreting thyroid stimulating hormone results in the diagnosis of thyroid dysfunction. J Thyroid Res. 2019;2019:4106816.
29. Skelin M, Lucijanić T, Amidžić Klarić D, et al. Factors affecting gastrointestinal absorption of levothyroxine: a review. Clin Ther. 2017;39:378–403.
30. Virili C, Antonelli A, Santaguida MG, Benvenga S, Centanni M. Gastrointestinal malabsorption of thyroxine. Endocr Rev. 2019;40:118–36.
31. Virili C, Trimboli P, Centanni M. Novel thyroxine formulations: a further step toward precision medicine. Endocrine. 2019;66:87–94.
32. Kumar R, Shaukat F. Adherence to levothyroxine tablet in patients with hypothyroidism. Cureus. 2019;11:e4624.
33. Gonzales KM, Stan MN, Morris JC 3rd, Bernet V, Castro MR. The levothyroxine absorption test: a four-year experience (2015-2018) at The Mayo Clinic. Thyroid. 2019;29:1734–42.
34. Garayalde Gamboa MLÁ, Saban M, Curriá MI. Treatment with intramuscular levothyroxine in refractory hypothyroidism. Eur Thyroid J. 2019;8:319–23.
35. Alexander EK, Pearce EN, Brent GA, et al. 2017 Guidelines of the American Thyroid Association for the diagnosis and management of thyroid disease during pregnancy and the postpartum. Thyroid. 2017;27:315–89.
36. Faix JD, Thienpoint LM. American Association of Clinical Chemists. Thyroid-stimulating hormone. Why efforts to harmonize testing are critical to patient care. Clinical Laboratory News. 2013. Available at https://www.aacc.org/publications/cln/articles/2013/may/tsh-harmonization. Accessed Jul 2019.

37. Koulouri O, Moran C, Halsall D, Chatterjee K, Gurnell M. Pitfalls in the measurement and interpretation of thyroid function tests. Best Pract Res Clin Endocrinol Metab. 2013;27:745–62.
38. Cappelli C, Rotondi M, Pirola I, et al. TSH-lowering effect of metformin in type 2 diabetic patients. Differences between euthyroid, untreated hypothyroid, and euthyroid on L-T4 therapy. Diabetes Care. 2009;32:1589–90.
39. Lupoli R, Di Minno A, Tortora A, Ambrosino P, Lupoli GA, Di Minno MN. Effects of treatment with metformin on TSH levels: a meta-analysis of literature studies. J Clin Endocrinol Metab. 2014;99:E143–8.
40. McMillan M, Rotenberg KS, Vora K, et al. Comorbidities, concomitant medications, and diet as factors affecting levothyroxine therapy: results of the CONTROL Surveillance Project. Drugs R D. 2016;16:53–68.
41. Warade J, Pandey A. Diurnal variation of TSH: factor affecting interpretation of test. J Pharm Biomed Sci. 2014;4:776–80.
42. Yoshihara A, Noh JY, Watanabe N, et al. Seasonal changes in serum thyrotropin concentrations observed from big data obtained during six consecutive years from 2010 to 2015 at a single hospital in Japan. Thyroid. 2018;28:429–36.
43. Ehrenkranz J, Bach PR, Snow GL, et al. Circadian and circannual rhythms in thyroid hormones: determining the TSH and free T4 reference intervals based upon time of day, age, and sex. Thyroid. 2015;25:954–61.
44. Hollowell JG, Staehling NW, Flanders WD, et al. Serum TSH, T(4), and thyroid antibodies in the United States population (1988 to 1994):National Health and Nutrition Examination Survey (NHANES III). J Clin Endocrinol Metab. 2002;87:489–99.
45. Kim SJ, Kim MJ, Yoon SG, et al. Impact of smoking on thyroid gland: dose-related effect of urinary cotinine levels on thyroid function and thyroid autoimmunity. Sci Rep. 2019;9:4213.
46. Sanyal D, Raychaudhuri M. Hypothyroidism and obesity: an intriguing link. Indian J Endocrinol Metab. 2016;20:554–7.
47. Biondi B. Thyroid and obesity: an intriguing relationship. J Clin Endocrinol Metab. 2010;95:3614–7.
48. Hattori N, Ishihara T, Shimatsu A. Variability in the detection of macro TSH in different immunoassay systems. Eur J Endocrinol. 2016;174:9–15.
49. Després N, Grant AM. Antibody interference in thyroid assays: a potential for clinical misinformation. Clin Chem. 1998;44:440–54.
50. European Medicines Agency. Committee for Proprietary medicinal Products (CPMP). Note for guidance on the investigation of bioavailability and bioequivalence. Available at http://www.ema.europa.eu/docs/en_GB/document_library/Scientific_guideline/2009/09/WC500003519.pdf. Accessed Jul 2020.
51. European Medicines Agency. Committee For Medicinal Products for Human Use (CHMP). Guideline on the investigation of bioequivalence. Doc. Ref.: CPMP/EWP/QWP/1401/98 Rev. 1, Jan 2010. Available at http://www.ema.europa.eu/docs/en_GB/document_library/Scientific_guideline/2010/01/WC500070039.pdf. Accessed Jul 2020.
52. Davit B, Braddy AC, Conner DP, Yu LX. International guidelines for bioequivalence of systemically available orally administered generic drug products: a survey of similarities and differences. AAPS J. 2013;15:974–90.
53. Medicines and Health Regulatory Authority. Levothyroxine tablet products: a review of clinical & quality considerations. 7 Jan 2013. Available at http://webarchive.nationalarchives.gov.uk/20141205150130/http:/www.mhra.gov.uk/home/groups/pl-p/documents/drugsafetymessage/con222566.pdf. Accessed Jul 2020.
54. Agence Française de Sécrurité Sanitaire des Produits de Santé 2012. Commission Nationale de Pharmacovigilance. Compte rendu de la réunion du mardi 27 Mars 2012. Available at https://ansm.sante.fr/var/ansm_site/storage/original/application/4e4d2a70e5dddfb150fe87360d6b13dd.pdf. Accessed Jul 2020.

55. The United States Pharmacopeial Convention. 2009. Current USP monograph of levothyroxine sodium tablets (published in Revision Bulletin, Official 1 Feb 2010). Available at https://www.uspnf.com/sites/default/files/usp_pdf/EN/USPNF/levothyroxineSodiumTablets.pdf. Accessed Jul 2020.
56. Lipp HP, Hostalek U. A new formulation of levothyroxine engineered to meet new specification standards. Curr Med Res Opin. 2019;35:147–50.

Pharmacodynamic and Therapeutic Actions of Levothyroxine

James V. Hennessey

The regulation of thyroid hormones within the hypothalamic-pituitary-thyroid axis is complex, consisting of multiple feedback and feed-forward loops. In addition, this system contributes to and likely reflects the regulation of sensitivity to thyroid hormones at the level of other target tissues. The effects of levothyroxine (LT4) replacement therapy for people with hypothyroidism must be considered within this context, as many patients will have residual thyroid activity. LT4 replacement reverses many metabolic disturbances associated with hypothyroidism including resetting of reduced energy expenditure and metabolic rate, correction of dyslipidaemia, improvement in insulin sensitivity and glycaemic control, and reversal of a pro-inflammatory and procoagulant state, and the eventual correction of mood disturbances (although on the surface these appear more refractory to LT4 treatment than other consequences of hypothyroidism). Monotherapy with LT4 remains the mainstay of treatment for hypothyroidism, due to a lack of clinical evidence for superior treatment outcomes with combinations of LT4 and triiodothyronine.

1 Introduction

The opening chapters of this book outlined the historical development of levothyroxine (LT4) as a treatment for hypothyroidism and described the pharmacokinetic properties of exogenously applied levothyroxine. The purpose of this chapter is to summarise the therapeutic actions of LT4 in key organs of the body. Exogenous

J. V. Hennessey (✉)
Harvard Medical School, Division of Endocrinology, Beth Israel Deaconess Medical Center, Boston, MA, USA
e-mail: jhenness@bidmc.harvard.edu

© The Author(s) 2021
G. J. Kahaly (ed.), *70 Years of Levothyroxine*,
https://doi.org/10.1007/978-3-030-63277-9_3

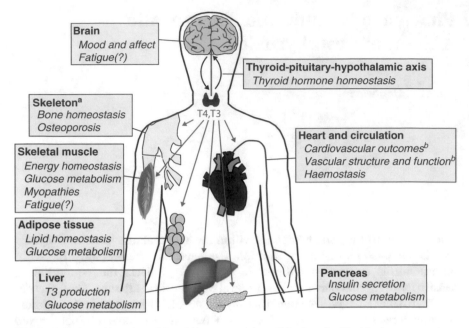

Fig. 1 Overview of key sites of thyroid hormone action. [a,b]Not described in this chapter: see chapters, "Levothyroxine and the Heart[a]" and "Levothyroxine and Bone[b]"

LT4 is indistinguishable from endogenous T4, and so I have sought to summarise the biological actions of T4 *per se*, in terms of the regulation of secretion and action of thyroid hormones and the therapeutic effects of LT4 supplementation in people with hypothyroidism in key areas of the body (Fig. 1). This chapter will not include detailed descriptions of the effects of LT4 on the heart or the skeleton: these aspects are covered in chapters, "Levothyroxine and the Heart" and "Levothyroxine and Bone" of this book, respectively. Finally, I have considered the evolution and current status of guidelines for the management of hypothyroidism, and the current evidence base for the therapeutic use of LT4 monotherapy, the current mainstay of treatment for hypothyroidism.

2 Thyroid Hormone Homeostasis

A simplistic view of the hypothalomo-pituitary-thyroid (HPT) axis entails secretion of thyrotropin-releasing hormone (TRH) from the hypothalamus acting on the pituitary to enhance secretion of thyrotropin (thyroid-stimulating hormone, TSH) [1–3]. Increased circulating concentrations of TSH then stimulate release of thyroid hormones from the thyroid gland, with a negative feedback loop causing secretion of TSH to fall as the concentration of thyroid hormones in the blood and tissues increases. In practice, the operation of the HPT axis is extraordinarily complex. Key components of the HPT, illustrating some of these complexities, are summarised below [3].

2.1 Conversion of T4 to T3

T4 is the primary secretory product of the thyroid and accounts for about 60–80% of circulating thyroid hormones. Triiodothyronine (T3) accounts for most of the remainder (other molecular species such as diiothyronine, or reverse T3 may have biological activity [4], but are beyond the scope of this review). Eighty percent of the T3 found in the circulation is derived through peripheral activation of T4 while the remaining 20% of circulating T3 is produced in the thyroid. T4 (or exogenous LT4) is converted to T3 locally in target tissues, via the actions of three deiodinase enzymes, particularly Deiodinase 2 (see chapter, "Administration and Pharmacokinetics of Levothyroxine" for a fuller account of the functions of different deiodinases) [5].

2.2 Regulation of Deiodinases and Individual "Set Points" for Thyroid Function

The activity of intrathyroidal deiodinase is regulated by TSH in a feed-forward manner, providing a means of adjustment of local T3 levels as needed [3]. In addition, ubiquitination of Deiodinase 2 in some tissues reduces its activity; this occurs to a lesser extent in the hypothalamus than in some other tissues, which may increase sensitivity to feedback inhibition of TRH release by (L)T4 [6].

The relationship between TSH levels, free T3 and free T4 (FT3 and FT4) is not the same in a euthyroid healthy individual and a patient with thyroid disease treated with LT4 [7, 8]. In general, T4 levels (especially when measured in the post-absorptive state) tend to be higher once TSH is controlled to its reference range, compared with euthyroid individuals [9–11]. However, studies in hypothyroid patients rendered surgically athyroid who were titrated to a normal TSH with LT4 have also reported normalised T3 levels; in fact, 49% of those titrated to a normal TSH had higher T3 levels on LT4 than in their native preoperative state in one study [12]. A retrospective study of hypothyroid subjects on LT4 monotherapy reported lower FT3 levels than in healthy individuals [13]. Finally, in one retrospective study, serum T3 levels in subjects with an elevated or normal-range TSH were lower than the same individuals' preoperative values but surprisingly all were still within the normal reference range. In those with modest TSH suppression, T3 levels were no different from their native state while several of those with more complete suppression of TSH demonstrated frankly elevated T3 values [8]. Accordingly, each patient with thyroid dysfunction has an individual "set point" for optimum functioning of the HPT axis, whether levels of TSH, FT3, and FT4 are precisely within their formally defined reference ranges or not [14].

2.3 Thyroid Hormone Receptors (THRs)

THRs are nuclear receptors that bind T3 after uptake into cells via active transporters. The most important THRs for mediating the actions of thyroid hormones are [13, 15, 16]:

- THRα1: expressed most strongly in bone, the gut, the central nervous system, and cardiac and skeletal muscle
- THRβ1: expressed most strongly in the liver, kidney, and the inner ear
- THRβ2: expressed most strongly in the hypothalamus, pituitary, cochlea, and retina

THRβ2 appears to be about ten-fold more sensitive than THRβ1 [13]. Loss-of-function mutations in THRs have been shown to produce elevated circulating T4 and T3 levels simultaneously with signs of a functional peripheral hypothyroidism [17].

2.4   Regulation of TSH Release

Production of TRH by the hypothalamus is an absolute requirement for the production of TSH, and thus thyroidal T4 [18]. TRH modulates the bioactivity of TSH, with more bioactive forms produced in the setting of thyroid deficiency [19]. TSH itself exerts an autocrine function in the pituitary and a paracrine function in the hypothalamus to inhibit further TSH release [20].

Importantly, TSH release is highly sensitive to the prevailing level of T4 in the circulation, such that reducing FT4 by half would typically increase the TSH level by up to 100-fold; conversely, a five-fold increase in the TSH level might be seen when FT4 is reduced by only about 10% [21]. The relationship of TSH levels to FT4 levels has been described as inverse log-linear although more complex non-linear associations have been described [22–25]. This relationship is the main reason why the TSH level is used to guide treatment of hypothyroidism with LT4, as the large changes in TSH are far easier to measure than small changes in T4 or FT4 (within the traditional 95% normal range) in the routine setting [21, 26]. Multiple factors, such as age, gender, smoking, the presence of antithyroid antibodies, and the difference between prevailing thyroid hormone levels and an individual's "set point" for HPT axis function (see above), influence the shape of the relationship between TSH and FT4 levels [22, 23, 25].

3   Clinical Pharmacodynamics of (Levo)Thyroxine

3.1   Which Thyroid Hormones Are Important?

LT4 acts essentially as a prodrug of T3 in target tissues, via the actions of the deiodinase enzymes, described above [5]. Accordingly, this section will include information on the effects of hypothyroidism on key organs of the body, as well as the restorative effects of treatment with LT4. Table 1 summarises these effects of LT4 replacement on important physiologic and metabolic processes in patients with hypothyroidism.

Table 1 Overview of the pharmacodynamics of LT4 in key physiological or organ systems in patients with hypothyroidism

Physiological process	Influence of hypothyroidism	Principal effects of LT4 replacement in a patient with hypothyroidism
Energy expenditure	Reduced	Reverses reductions in resting energy expenditure and metabolic rate
Lipid profiles	Promotes dyslipidaemia mainly via ↓ hepatic LDL receptors	Reduces total and LDL-cholesterol, and other markers of dyslipidaemia Reduces intrahepatic lipid content (where elevated)
Blood glucose control	Overt hypothyroidism mitigates IGT Subclinical hypothyroidism increases insulin resistance and risk of diabetes	Corrects changes of IGT in thyrotoxicosis Improves insulin sensitivity Improves glucose tolerance
Inflammation	Increased systemic inflammation	Reduced markers of systemic inflammation
Coagulation[a]	Overt hypocoagulant state often induces coagulopathy similar to aVWS Subclinical hypothyroidism induces a procoagulant state	LT4 corrects deficiencies Improved markers of fibrinolysis and coagulation
Brain	Altered mood/affect	Evidence for improved mood/affect (e.g. reduced depression questionnaire scores)
Adipose tissue	Modest ↑ weight ↓ Brown fat activation	Reverses weight gain in hypothyroidism (but little effect on body composition)
Heart[a]	Exacerbates existing cardiac issues Reduced cardiac contractility Increased blood pressure	Reverses abnormalities in cardiac structure and function
Bone[a]	Thyroid hormones reduce bone density	Over treatment and hyperthyroidism may cause excessive bone loss Thyroid function must be assessed especially carefully in people at risk of fractures
Kidney	Hypothyroidism can reduce renal function	Reverses hypothyroidism-induced reduction in GFR Some evidence of benefit (reduced decline in GFR, reduced uric acid and albumin excretion)
QoL	Decreased health-related QoL Fatigue is common	Inconsistent effects of LT4 on relatively non-specific symptoms (importance of ensuring an accurate diagnosis of hypothyroidism)

[a]Dealt with only briefly here, see chapters, "Levothyroxine and the Heart" and "Levothyroxine and Bone" of this book for a fuller account of the effects of hypothyroidism and LT4 on these organs, including discussion of the effects on cardiac outcomes. *aVWS* acquired Von Willebrand Syndrome, *GFR* glomerular filtration rate, *IGT* impaired glucose tolerance, *QoL* quality of life. See text for references

3.2   Actions on Skeletal Muscle

3.2.1   Mechanisms

Skeletal muscle is a major site of action of thyroid hormones. Active membrane transporters regulate the uptake of T4 and T3 from the extracellular space; once inside the cell, the T3 level is adjusted via deiodination of T4 and inactivation of T3, by Deiodinases 2 and 3, respectively [27–29]. Activation of the thyroid receptor drives multiple processes, from the initiation of muscle formation during early embryogenesis, to the differentiation of the various fast and slow skeletal muscle fibre phenotypes in adult muscle (high T3 levels favour fast-twitch type muscle fibres [30]), to the repair or replacement of damaged muscle fibres [27, 28]. Defects in these mechanisms, associated with changes in levels of thyroid hormones, may be implicated in the progression of myopathy states, including Duchenne muscular dystrophy, among others [31]. High levels of thyroid hormones increase energy utilisation, and decrease the efficiency of skeletal muscle, with opposite effects in hypothyroidism. Skeletal muscle accounts for up to half of an individual's body weight and changes in energy homeostasis in skeletal muscle exert an important influence on the overall metabolic rate [27, 28].

3.2.2   Clinical Studies of Interest

LT4 replacement therapy vs. no treatment has been shown to improve cardiopulmonary performance (O_2 uptake, minute ventilation, and heart rate) in subjects with subclinical hypothyroidism [32], although not all studies have shown this [33]. In another study, variation of LT4 doses to induce minor fluctuations of TSH around the reference range did not influence energy expenditure or body composition in patients with hypothyroidism [34]. Studies in euthyroid subjects showed variable effects of LT4 on muscle performance [35–37], consistent with the absence of indications for LT4 intervention in those without hypothyroidism.

3.3   Effects on Lipid Profiles

Thyroid hormones are metabolised in the liver, which influences their levels in the circulation [38]. T3 in the liver induces 3-hydroxy-3-methylglutaryl-coenzyme A (HMG-CoA, which initiates cholesterol synthesis), increases the synthesis and release of LDL receptors (enhancing LDL-cholesterol clearance), and stimulates the activity of lipoprotein lipase and apolipoprotein AV (which play a major role in triglyceride regulation) [39]. Thus, even mild hypothyroidism increases total cholesterol, LDL-cholesterol and, sometimes, triglycerides [40]. The administration of LT4 reduces serum cholesterol and other markers of dyslipidaemia in patients with varying degrees of hypothyroidism [40–44]. LT4 also reduced intrahepatic lipid content in an uncontrolled study in euthyroid subjects with non-alcoholic fatty liver disease and type 2 diabetes, suggesting a possible future role for LT4 in this population [45]. At present, LT4 does not have a recognised role in dyslipidaemia management of euthyroid individuals, however [46].

3.4 Actions in Adipose Tissue

Thyroid hormones have a powerful effect in stimulating thermogenesis in brown adipose tissue, to a much greater extent than that observed in white adipose tissue [27, 47]. TSH correlates positively with body mass index, and overt hypothyroidism is associated with modest weight gain, which reverses with LT4 treatment; however, this weight loss may be associated more with loss of excess fluid than loss of fat mass [48]. A study in women with hypothyroidism showed that normalisation of TSH with LT4 did not affect body fat percentage significantly [49]. Changes in resting energy expenditure during LT4 treatment in humans are driven mainly by effects in skeletal muscle, as described above.

3.5 Effects on Glucose Metabolism

An association of autoimmune thyroid disease and type 1 diabetes mellitus has long been recognised [50, 51]. Thyrotoxicosis was long believed to be the prime thyroid function abnormality associated with glucose intolerance and two-thirds of those found to be glucose intolerant while thyrotoxic were normal when retested after adequate antithyroid treatment; on the other hand, glucose intolerance persisted in the remainder [52]. Increased intestinal hexose absorption, decreased responsiveness to insulin, and increased glucose production have been proposed to mediate hyperglycaemic effects of thyrotoxicosis [50]. Further observations of insulin secretion/action defects in thyrotoxicosis were mainly accounted for by ageing [53, 54]. Normal insulin secretory function and adipocyte sensitivity in the face of a reduced number of adipocyte insulin receptors shifted the search for a mechanism toward the hepatocyte and resultant increased gluconeogenesis or changes in skeletal muscle glucose metabolism as the basis of glucose intolerance in thyrotoxic patients [55–57]. In summary, an increase in T3 activity as seen in overt hyperthyroidism, seems to drive increased production of glucose by the liver and may be associated with reduced insulin secretion from the pancreas, increasing the risk of glucose intolerance and diabetes [27].

Ironically, more recent research indicates that overt thyrotoxicosis is not necessarily the only influence on glucose intolerance and frank type 2 diabetes in genetically at-risk subjects. In fact, compared with euglycaemic, unrelated controls, those with new onset type 2 diabetes, impaired glucose intolerance (IGT) and relatives of type 2 diabetes patients had higher FT4 and FT3 though all were within the expected range [58]. Cross-sectional observations showed that impaired fasting glucose (IFG) was associated with higher free T3 and FT3/FT4 ratios but lower FT4 than IGT, indicating that thyroid hormone levels may play differing roles in the development of different forms of dysglycaemia [59]. Further evidence of a direct influence of inadequate

Fig. 2 Overview of some
important effects of
levothyroxine on
glycaemia. [a]Effects
mediated via decreased
apoptosis and enhanced
growth and differentiation.
(Compiled from
information presented in
Ref. [51])

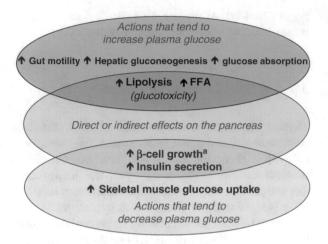

thyroid function on insulin resistance was reported in a group of athyrotic subjects, in the form of a negative correlation of FT4 and insulin during thyroid hormone withdrawal [60]. Another study showed that people with overt and subclinical hypothyroidism had similar severity of insulin resistance, each higher than in euthyroid controls, providing further evidence that hypothyroidism is an insulin-resistant state [61]. A study of 2,399 euthyroid, non-diabetic subjects showed that FT4 levels in the lower part of the normal range were associated with an increased risk of prediabetes [62], and other clinical data indicated that higher TSH levels, as found in hypothyroidism, increase the risk of developing type 2 diabetes [63].

Correction of subclinical hypothyroidism with LT4 has been shown to improve insulin resistance and/or control of blood glucose [42, 64–66]. A recent study showed that malabsorption of LT4 associated with concomitant calcium carbonate supplementation was associated with a decline in the quality of glycaemic control, which was reversed when the interval between LT4 and calcium supplementation was increased [67]. Practically, and reassuringly, exogenous LT4 does not seem to be associated with glucose tolerance issues, even at TSH-suppressive doses that result in prolonged subclinical thyrotoxicosis [68].

These studies leave us with some unanswered questions in regard to the mechanisms linking thyroid function and glucose intolerance. A recent review summarises six areas of mechanistic connections between the presence of thyrotoxicosis and abnormal glucose metabolism, and Fig. 2 summarises its main findings [51].

3.6   Actions on Mood and Affect

The hypothalamus is involved intimately in the complex relationships between thyroid hormone status and numerous aspects of metabolism and homeostasis, as described above. Changes in mood and affect are classically recognised symptoms of hypothyroidism [69]. LT4 administration to symptomatic hypothyroid subjects should improve mood and affect only if thyroid function provoked such symptoms.

Unfortunately, recent observations in subclinical thyroid dysfunction alert us to the need to diagnose specific underlying thyroid abnormalities accurately, rather than empirically assuming a thyroid-deficient state. Subclinical hyperthyroidism has emerged as a more frequent underpinning of depression than mild thyroid failure [70–72], indicating that thyroid hormone replacement would not be universally appropriate for all situations where hypothyroidism is assumed to be present. Although some studies have reported very robust improvement in thyroid-specific symptoms when LT4 is used to titrate TSH into the normal range [73, 74], and other investigations seem to indicate that LT4 treated patients fare as well as appropriately selected controls [75], some investigators emphasise less than perfect resolution of symptoms with thyroid hormone replacement therapies [76–78].

Recently, a randomised, placebo-controlled trial in 60 patients with subclinical hypothyroidism did demonstrate a significant improvement in Beck Depression Inventory (BDI) scores in those randomised to LT4 therapy, while improvement was not observed in the placebo group [79]. The effect in the LT4 group was driven strongly by improvements in the somatic subscale of the BDI, with no significant improvement in the affect scale. A case-control study indicated that a population of women with hypothyroidism continued to have a higher prevalence of anxiety or depression than a control group of euthyroid women, even after correction of TSH using LT4 [80]. These findings have prompted some experts to propose individually derived cut-offs for TSH in the management of hypothyroidism with LT4, that is based on resolution of symptoms of depression [81]. These contradictory findings emphasise the current difficulties encountered in identifying specific symptoms truly due to thyroid hormone deficiency rather than the other, common, non-thyroid-related, symptoms that result in a major obstacle in the clinical assessment of self-reported complaints, especially in patients with chronic conditions [82]. Such symptoms would not be expected to respond to manipulation of the thyroid axis in those with normal thyroid function. Multiple alternative explanations for LT4-treated subjects' occasional unhappiness with their clinical outcomes have been reported extensively and potentially include independent effects of autoimmunity [83, 84], theoretical brain hypothyroidism with normal TSH [85], selection bias of subjects seeking health care [86], and awareness of having a chronic disease [87]. These and other explanations will be discussed in detail below.

Some have speculated that the documentation of biochemical hypothyroidism is less sensitive than clinical symptoms in identifying truly hypothyroid individuals who would benefit from LT4 replacement therapy. These anecdotal and testimonial reports seldom acknowledge the lack of effect of LT4 vs. placebo on the Hospital Anxiety/Depression Scale (HADS) and the Standard Form-36 (SF-36) in a randomised trial [88]. It seems clear that symptoms consistent with hypothyroidism in euthyroid individuals do not respond to (nor should they be treated with) LT4.

The relationship between hypothyroidism and the response of neuropsychiatric function to LT4 therapy has continued to generate interest in the potential application of LT4 treatment to correct these symptoms in euthyroid patients with psychiatric disorders. One study did not find a significant effect of LT4 on a validated instrument for quantifying symptoms of depression in people with bipolar disorder [89], while randomised [90] or observational [91] trials have indicated improved mood in euthyroid patients with bipolar disorder given an LT4 300 µg/day. It is difficult to disassociate effects on mood of LT4 *per se* from the adverse psychological impact of having a chronic thyroid condition, however [92]. LT4 is not indicated for this purpose, and these studies remain in the realm of research.

3.7 Fatigue

Patients with fatigue (a classic symptom of hypothyroidism) are reported to receive a lifetime diagnosis of depression or anxiety disorder much more frequently than others (45% vs. 28%) [93]. Similarly, tiredness, another non-specific "thyroid" symptom common in primary care is associated as frequently with chronic diseases such as diabetes, or anaemia, as with hypothyroidism, and more strongly associated with depression [94]. The correlation of symptoms consistent with hypothyroidism and actual, documentable hypothyroidism is poor [95]. The predictive value of individual symptoms in identifying hypothyroidism is substantially overlapping with symptoms offered by euthyroid individuals [96], and this lack of specificity is diminished even further by female gender and older age [97]. Persistent symptoms encountered in those on thyroid hormone replacement with well-controlled TSH levels and normal serum T3 levels have been demonstrated to be correlated more closely with comorbidities than thyroid function [98, 99], again highlighting the importance of assessing the entire patient rather than to assume that all complaints are thyroid related.

3.8 Actions on Inflammation and Haemostasis

Circulating levels of inflammatory cytokines were increased in hypothyroidism and reduced after treatment with LT4 in a randomised, placebo-controlled trial [100] and in an observational study [101]. In general, low levels of circulating thyroid hormone shift the haemostatic system to a hypocoagulable hyper-fibrinolytic state, with reduced Factors VIII, IX, and XI and von Willebrand factor (VWF) that are normalised on LT4 [102, 103]. The coagulopathy of overt hypothyroidism has been referred to as an acquired von Willebrand syndrome (aVWS), seen in about one-third of these patients, with low VWF and FIII, with mucocutaneous bleeding that responds to desmopressin [104–106]. The incidence of aVWS may approach 33% of those with overt hypothyroidism, may play a role of the menorrhagia observed in hypothyroidism, and may diminish the risk of venous thromboembolism (VTE) [105, 106]. Subclinical hypothyroidism is paradoxically associated with a shift to a procoagulant state, with higher FVII, PAI-1, and tissue plasminogen activator (t-PA), which seem to normalise with 6 months of LT4 [107]. Thrombin-activatable fibrinolysis inhibitor (TAFI) levels are elevated, and global fibrinolytic capacity is lower, vs. control subjects in subclinical hypothyroidism [108, 109]. Correction of TSH levels to normal using LT4 replacement correct these abnormalities [102, 110, 111].

Excess thyroid hormone activity results in a procoagulant state, with increased VWF, FVIII, fibrinogen, and D-dimer in subclinical hyperthyroidism and elevations in fibrinogen, fibronectin, VWF, thrombomodulin, and PAI-1, with decreased t-PA in overt, endogenous hyperthyroidism [103, 112–115]. The enhanced risk of VTE (deep vein thrombosis or pulmonary embolism) has been expertly summarised recently [103]. This underlying prothrombotic state interacts with the additional risk of atrial fibrillation/flutter to elevate the risk of ischaemic stroke [116]. Underlying mechanisms may include the presence of autoimmune disease, but unique observations from subjects with thyroid hormone resistance at the TRβ infer that the hyper-coagulation seen in thyrotoxicosis is a direct consequence of T3 action on levels of the coagulation factors described above [117]. Thyrotoxicosis induced by administration of LT4 to healthy volunteers and those with thyroid nodules also induces a procoagulant state, associated with increased levels of FVIII, FIX, FX, VWF, fibrinogen D-dimer, and PAI-1 with delayed fibrin clot lysis and a shortening of the APTT, but with an inconsistent impact on clot structure parameters potentially based on subtle mechanistic differences between endogenous and iatrogenic hyperthyroidism [118–121].

3.9 Effects in the Kidney

The hypothyroid state itself reduces renal function [122]. Administration of LT4 has been observed to improve renal function, in one study improving odds of progression and lowering the incidence of end-stage kidney disease by limiting the rate of decline in glomerular filtration rate [123]. In another randomised, placebo-controlled study, LT4 treatment reduced serum uric acid and excretion of albumin in a trial in patients with diabetic nephropathy and subclinical hypothyroidism, an effect consistent with a renoprotective effect [41].

3.10 Effects on the Heart and in Bone

Chapters, "Levothyroxine and the Heart" and "Levothyroxine and Bone" provide a description of the effects of LT4 in heart and bone, and only a brief summary is provided here in Table 1.

4 Evidence-Based Guidelines for the Management of Hypothyroidism

4.1 Current Status of Evidence-Based Guidelines

The American Thyroid Association (ATA) has been publishing regular guidance on the management of thyroid disease since its recommendations on nomenclature for goitre in 1931 [124]. The most recent ATA guideline for the management of hypothyroidism (2014) considered 64 questions relating to the care of these patients, grouped under 24 topics [125]. An overview of its strong recommendations with regard to the management of overt hypothyroidism in adults is given in Table 2.

Table 2 Summary of "strong" recommendations relating to the management of overt hypothyroidism from a guideline proposed by the American Thyroid Association

Main therapy	Monotherapy with LT4 adjusted using TSH; thyroid extracts are not recommended.
Key goals of therapy	Normalise TSH (and improve other thyroid hormones), abolish symptoms (including lipid abnormalities), avoid over treatment (iatrogenic thyrotoxicosis).
Starting dose	Consider factors including weight, age, comorbidity, aetiology of thyroid disease, starting TSH, desired TSH goal when deciding on starting LT4 dose.
Mental health/ behavioural issues	Consider a mental health professional if psychosocial, behavioural, or mental health symptoms do not respond adequately to LT4, or if these issues impair management.
Elderly patients	Start with low dose, increase slowly (NB: ideal TSH may be higher in older patients).
Pregnancy	Use trimester-specific TSH reference ranges to guide therapy.[a]
Infants	Treat as soon as hypothyroidism is confirmed; aim to move TSH to the mid-to-lower half of the paediatric TSH reference range within 2–4 weeks.
Subgroups/ comorbidities	There is no evidence to support targeting low- or high-normal TSH for subgroups such as those with obesity, depression, dyslipidaemia, or no thyroid function.
Secondary hypothyroidism	Maintain the FT4 in the upper half of the reference range (may be lower in older patients or those with comorbidities).
Well-being and quality of life	Use general instruments + hypothyroidism-specific tools to evaluate general well-being and quality of life during treatment.
Euthyroid subjects	Do not use LT4 in biochemically euthyroid people with hypothyroid-like symptoms or for the management of obesity, depression, urticaria, or dyslipidaemia
Thyroid hormone abuse	Withdraw thyroid hormones from patients with factitious thyrotoxicosis and refer for education and/or psychological support
LT4 + T3 therapy	Insufficient clinical evidence to support a routine-use recommendation[b]
Nutraceuticals and supplements	Not supported in hypothyroidism management (pharmacological doses of iodine may exacerbate underlying thyroid pathology)
Hospitalised/not critically ill patients	Consider starting or adjusting oral LT4 (consider temporary use of i.v. LT4 if necessary), based on normalisation of TSH; exclude adrenal insufficiency
Myxoedema coma	Start with i.v. LT4 (+standard management for coma including glucocorticoids), with starting dose depending on age and comorbidities, and switch to oral LT4 when possible. Improved mental status and improved cardiac/pulmonary function are key early measurements, follow thyroid hormones thereafter
"Nonthyroidal illness syndrome"	LT4 is not recommended for hospitalised patients with this condition.

Recommendations are abstracted from Ref. [125]. They have been paraphrased for brevity, and combined in some cases. Only strong recommendations relating to the use of LT4 are included here: see the full guideline for details

[a]See chapter, "Levothyroxine in Pregnancy" for a description of hypothyroidism management in pregnancy. *GI* gastrointestinal, *LT4* levothyroxine, *TSH* thyrotropin, thyroid-stimulating hormone

[b]Evidence for LT4 + T3 combination therapy is discussed later in this chapter

These guidelines emphasise the key role of monotherapy with LT4 (the use of thyroid extracts is not supported) in the management of hypothyroidism, due mainly to its proven efficacy and safety profile, long half-life and low cost. The level of thyrotropin is used to guide therapy in almost all circumstances, rather than other thyroid hormones, or symptoms of hypothyroidism. The therapeutic use of LT4 for other conditions, such as obesity, psychiatric conditions, and dyslipidaemia, is not supported and such uses remain an area for research (see above). A guideline from the UK National Institute for Health and Care Excellence (2019) provided similar recommendations [126].

The 2014 ATA guidance did not address the issue of managing subclinical hypothyroidism. Additional information is now available from the TRUST study, a large, prospective, randomised, controlled trial of LT4 in a population likely to be enriched with people with subclinical hypothyroidism (TSH >4.6 mIU/L with normal FT4) [127]. A total of 737 patients aged >65 years were recruited and the primary outcome parameter was QoL (Thyroid-Related Quality of Life Patient Reported Outcome [ThyPro] subscales for hypothyroid symptoms score and tiredness score). Neither thyroid symptoms nor tiredness scores were changed significantly in the LT4 or placebo groups by 12 months [127]. Reassuringly, there were no adverse effects of LT4. Although the quality of this trial warranted publication in a premier medical journal, the use of non-age-adjusted TSH at entry likely led to the inclusion of many functionally euthyroid subjects, rendering demonstration of a therapeutic effect of LT4 very unlikely. Although the TSH levels in those on LT4 were reduced impressively, one-quarter of subjects were asymptomatic. The mean baseline TSH in both groups was below the age expected 97.5th percentile (normal) of euthyroid, antibody negative individuals observed for the US population [128]. Additionally, the TSH levels of the placebo group had also normalised in an unknown but significant portion with no intervention, further reducing the potential for demonstrating a therapeutic impact of LT4.

A recent (2018), high quality meta-analysis of 21 randomised, placebo-controlled trials of LT4 ($N = 2192$ subclinically hypothyroid adults) focussed on QoL and thyroid-related symptoms and confirmed a lack of improvement with LT4 in these subjective endpoints [129]. A guideline from the European Thyroid Association (ETA) based on this meta-analysis recommended that a trial of LT4 should be considered in younger (<65 years) subjects with symptoms reminiscent of hypothyroidism with TSH that is elevated, but <10 mIU/L [130]. LT4 can be withdrawn if symptoms have not resolved after normalisation of the thyrotropin level. Younger subjects with thyrotropin >10 mIU/L should receive LT4 whether or not they have symptoms [130]. Another international expert group concluded that few patients with subclinical hypothyroidism would be likely to benefit from treatment with LT4 [131].

Another meta-analysis and independent review provided guidance on the need for confirmation of the diagnosis of mild thyroid failure/subclinical hypothyroidism in non-pregnant adults [132]. TSH and FT4 should be re-measured in 1–3 months when TSH is 4.5–14.9 mIU/L, and in 1–2 weeks when TSH is ≥15 mIU/L. Confirmation of the elevated TSH is considered essential in establishing the diagnosis of subclinical hypothyroidism although this is not a guarantee of persistent thyroid failure [127, 133]. Additionally, LT4 may be *considered* for reduced risk of progression to overt hypothyroidism and adverse cardiovascular outcomes for patients aged >65 years with TSH >7 mIU/L, and *offered* when TSH is persistently over 10 mIU/L. Recommendations for individuals aged <65 years are more liberal and recommend measurement of anti-TPO antibodies when the TSH is 4.5–6.9 mIU/L, with annual follow-up. LT4 treatment would be considered when multiple symptoms are present, TPO antibodies are positive, TSH is increasing, pregnancy is anticipated, or goitre is present. LT4 therapy is recommended in this age group when TSH is persistently >7.0 mIU/L [132].

4.2   Levothyroxine Monotherapy, or Levothyroxine Plus Triiodothyronine, for Hypothyroidism

Loss-of-function polymorphisms in deiodinases have been proposed to contribute to failure of thyrotropin-guided LT4 therapy to completely abolish symptoms of hypothyroidism in some patients, due to insufficient provision of T3 [134, 135]. This has stimulated interest (and use to this day) in LT4-levotriiodothyronine (liothyronine, LT3) combination therapy, or thyroid extracts (which are not supported by any guidelines), in these patients [135, 136]. The results of trials comparing LT4–LT3 combinations with LT4 monotherapy, or meta-analyses of these trials, have been inconsistent, without demonstrating convincing or consistent benefit for combination therapy [135, 137, 138]. In addition, the short plasma half-life of LT3 (hours), compared with that of LT4 (days) does not support straightforward once-daily administration of these combinations. Accordingly, there is currently no accepted role for the use of LT3 in the management of hypothyroidism [125, 135, 137].

It has been suggested that more trials are needed, in patients with reduced sensitivity to thyroid hormones [137]. Alternatively, differences in initial residual thyroid function between patients may have introduced variability into the results of these trials [139]. Although there is support in a European guideline for a trial of LT4-LT3 therapy in individuals with persistent hypothyroid-like symptoms on LT4 after exclusion of other possible causes [140], further research will be needed before this approach becomes part of the routine care of hypothyroidism.

4.3 Barriers to Optimal Care of Patients with Hypothyroidism

4.3.1 The Impact of the Diagnosis Itself

Diagnostic labelling influences individual patient's self-reported health results as illustrated in a recent report derived from the HUNT study which asked subjects to rate their perception of their health [141]. Data on thyroid function at entry were available to researchers only. Most (at least 75%) of the general population and subjects unaware of their thyroid dysfunction reported their health as good; however, only half of those aware of a diagnosis of thyroid dysfunction reported good health. Increasing age, lower education, smoking, low self-esteem, underweight, overweight, or obese and long-term illness/injury—but not thyroid function—predicted lower self-reported health.

4.3.2 Avoiding over Diagnosis

Who would typically be evaluated with thyroid function testing in a primary care practice and potentially labelled as hypothyroid? According to a study in the primary care setting, those referred for thyroid function tests have high rates of psychological stress and low (no) correlation of typical thyroid symptoms and thyroid test results [142]. The authors expressed concern that a mild TSH elevation might result in reflexive LT4 initiation. This of course assumes that the symptoms are truly due to hypothyroidism and a search for alternative explanations ends. I would point out that failure of LT4 intervention to cure these likely *non-thyroid* symptoms would not only disappoint our now-labelled patient, but might also distract the treating physician from the potential of psychiatric morbidity and initiate a quest for alternative thyroid solutions rather than providing the patient with the help they really need.

Once confidence in a diagnosis of hypothyroidism is established, further attempts to satisfy subjects treated with LT4 who continue to report symptoms consistent with hypothyroidism has led to the practice of finely titrating the TSH into specific tertiles of the expected range with small LT4 dose adjustments. Two excellent prospective controlled studies have used validated measures of health-related quality of life (HR-QoL) and cognition to demonstrate little or no benefit from this approach [143, 144]. Most importantly, patients were unable to correctly identify whether they had received the lower, medium, or higher dose, but associated the higher dose with a perception of greater efficacy [144].

5   Conclusions

Thyroid hormones are tightly integrated within the development, homeostasis, and repair of numerous tissues in the body, including the regulation of the HPT axis itself. Accordingly, hypothyroidism disturbs multiple functions within the body. Hormone replacement with LT4 can reverse many symptoms of hypothyroidism, including reduced energy expenditure, dyslipidaemia, and disturbances of diverse functions, including haemostasis and mood. Not all patients feel completely well on optimised LT4 therapy, however, often for various non-thyroid-related reasons. Variations in sensitivity to thyroid hormones, arising for example, in variations in genes for the deiodinases that convert LT4 to T3 within target tissues or in thyroid hormone transporters, may contribute to this phenomenon, and this remains a subject for future research. Monotherapy with LT4, optimised according to a normalised serum TSH level, remains the preferred treatment for hypothyroidism recommended by current major guidelines in this area.

References

1. Pirahanchi Y, Jialal I. Physiology, thyroid stimulating hormone (TSH). StatPearls [Internet]. Available at https://www.ncbi.nlm.nih.gov/books/NBK499850/. Accessed Jul 2020.
2. Mariotti S, Beck-Peccoz P. Physiology of the hypothalamic-pituitary-thyroid axis. Endotext [Internet]. Available at https://www.ncbi.nlm.nih.gov/books/NBK278958/. Accessed Jul 2020.
3. Hoermann R. Homeostatic control of the thyroid-pituitary axis: perspectives for diagnosis and treatment. Front Endocrinol (Lausanne). Nov 2015. Available at https://www.frontiersin.org/articles/10.3389/fendo.2015.00177/full. Accessed Jul 2020
4. Köhrle J. The colorful diversity of thyroid hormone metabolites. Eur Thyroid J. 2019;8:115–29.
5. Bianco AC, da Conceição RR. The deiodinase trio and thyroid hormone signaling. Methods Mol Biol. 2018;1801:67–83.
6. Werneck de Castro JP, Fonseca TL, Ueta CB, et al. Differences in hypothalamic type 2 deiodinase ubiquitination explain localized sensitivity to thyroxine. J Clin Invest. 2015;125:769–81.
7. Gullo D, Latina A, Frasca F, Le Moli R, Pellegriti G, Vigneri R. Levothyroxine monotherapy cannot guarantee euthyroidism in all athyreotic patients. PLoS One. 2011;6:e22552.
8. Ito M, Miyauchi A, Morita S, et al. TSH-suppressive doses of levothyroxine are required to achieve preoperative native serum triiodothyronine levels in patients who have undergone total thyroidectomy. Eur J Endocrinol. 2012;167:373–8.
9. Hennessey JV, Evaul JE, Tseng YC, Burman KD, Wartofsky L. L-thyroxine dosage: a reevaluation of therapy with contemporary preparations. Ann Intern Med. 1986;105:11–5.
10. Fish LH, Schwartz HL, Cavanaugh J, Steffes MW, Bantle JP, Oppenheimer JH. Replacement dose, metabolism, and bioavailability of levothyroxine in the treatment of hypothyroidism. Role of triiodothyronine in pituitary feedback in humans. N Engl J Med. 1987;316:764–70.
11. Liewendahl K, Helenius T, Lamberg BA, Mähönen H, Wägar G. Free thyroxine, free triiodothyronine, and thyrotropin concentrations in hypothyroid and thyroid carcinoma patients receiving thyroxine therapy. Acta Endocrinol (Copenh). 1987;116:418–24.
12. Jonklaas J, Davidson B, Bhagat S, Soldin SJ. Triiodothyronine levels in athyreotic individuals during levothyroxine therapy. JAMA. 2008;299:769–77.

13. Hoermann R, Midgley JE, Larisch R, Dietrich JW. Integration of peripheral and glandular regulation of triiodothyronine production by thyrotropin in untreated and thyroxine-treated subjects. Horm Metab Res. 2015;47:674–80.
14. Leow MK, Goede SL. The homeostatic set point of the hypothalamus-pituitary-thyroid axis—maximum curvature theory for personalized euthyroid targets. Theor Biol Med Model. 2014;11:35.
15. Anyetei-Anum CS, Roggero VR, Allison LA. Thyroid hormone receptor localization in target tissues. J Endocrinol. 2018;237:R19–34.
16. Ortiga-Carvalho TM, Sidhaye AR, Wondisford FE. Thyroid hormone receptors and resistance to thyroid hormone disorders. Nat Rev Endocrinol. 2014;10:582–91.
17. Singh BK, Yen PM. A clinician's guide to understanding resistance to thyroid hormone due to receptor mutations in the TRα and TRβ isoforms. Clin Diab Endocrinol. 2017;3:8.
18. Nikrodhanond AA, Ortiga-Carvalho TM, Shibusawa N, et al. Dominant role of thyrotropin-releasing hormone in the hypothalamic-pituitary-thyroid axis. J Biol Chem. 2006;281:5000–7.
19. Menezes-Ferreira MM, Petrick PA, Weintraub BD. Regulation of thyrotropin (TSH) bioactivity by TSH-releasing hormone and thyroid hormone. Endocrinology. 1986;118:2125–30.
20. Prummel MF, Brokken LJ, Wiersinga WM. Ultra short-loop feedback control of thyrotropin secretion. Thyroid. 2004;14:825–9.
21. Sheehan MT. Biochemical testing of the thyroid: TSH is the best and, oftentimes, only test needed—a review for primary care. Clin Med Res. 2016;14:83–92.
22. Brown SJ, Bremner AP, Hadlow NC, et al. The log TSH-free T4 relationship in a community-based cohort is nonlinear and is influenced by age, smoking and thyroid peroxidase antibody status. Clin Endocrinol (Oxf). 2016;85:789–96.
23. Hoermann R, Eckl W, Hoermann C, Larisch R. Complex relationship between free thyroxine and TSH in the regulation of thyroid function. Eur J Endocrinol. 2010;162:1123–9.
24. Rothacker KM, Brown SJ, Hadlow NC, Wardrop R, Walsh JP. Reconciling the log-linear and non-log-linear nature of the tsh-free t4 relationship: intra-individual analysis of a large population. J Clin Endocrinol Metab. 2016;101:1151–8.
25. Clark PM, Holder RL, Haque SM, Hobbs FD, Roberts LM, Franklyn JA. The relationship between serum TSH and free T4 in older people. Postgrad Med J. 2012;88:668–70.
26. Razvi S, Bhana S, Mrabeti S. Challenges in interpreting thyroid stimulating hormone results in the diagnosis of thyroid dysfunction. J Thyroid Res. 2019;2019:4106816.
27. Cicatiello AG, Di Girolamo D, Dentice M. Metabolic effects of the intracellular regulation of thyroid hormone: old players, new concepts. Front Endocrinol (Lausanne). 2018;9:474.
28. Salvatore D, Simonides WS, Dentice M, Zavacki AM, Larsen PR. Thyroid hormones and skeletal muscle—new insights and potential implications. Nat Rev Endocrinol. 2014;10:206–14.
29. Marsili A, Tang D, Harney JW, et al. Type II iodothyronine deiodinase provides intracellular 3,5,3'-triiodothyronine to normal and regenerating mouse skeletal muscle. Am J Physiol Endocrinol Metab. 2011;301:E818–24.
30. Larsson L, Li X, Teresi A, Salviati G. Effects of thyroid hormone on fast- and slow-twitch skeletal muscles in young and old rats. J Physiol. 1994;481:149–61.
31. Bloise FF, Oliveira TS, Cordeiro A, Ortiga-Carvalho TM. Thyroid hormones play role in sarcopenia and myopathies. Front Physiol. 2018;9:560.
32. Mainenti MR, Vigário PS, Teixeira PF, Maia MD, Oliveira FP, Vaisman M. Effect of levothyroxine replacement on exercise performance in subclinical hypothyroidism. J Endocrinol Investig. 2009;32:470–3.
33. Caraccio N, Natali A, Sironi A, et al. Muscle metabolism and exercise tolerance in subclinical hypothyroidism: a controlled trial of levothyroxine. J Clin Endocrinol Metab. 2005;90:4057–62.
34. Samuels MH, Kolobova I, Niederhausen M, Purnell JQ, Schuff KG. Effects of altering levothyroxine dose on energy expenditure and body composition in subjects treated with LT4. J Clin Endocrinol Metab. 2018;103:4163–75.

35. Rosenbaum M, Goldsmith RL, Haddad F, et al. Triiodothyronine and leptin repletion in humans similarly reverse weight-loss-induced changes in skeletal muscle. Am J Physiol Endocrinol Metab. 2018;315:E771–9.
36. Johannsen DL, Galgani JE, Johannsen NM, Zhang Z, Covington JD, Ravussin E. Effect of short-term thyroxine administration on energy metabolism and mitochondrial efficiency in humans. PLoS One. 2012;7:e40837.
37. Dubois S, Abraham P, Rohmer V, et al. Thyroxine therapy in euthyroid patients does not affect body composition or muscular function. Thyroid. 2008;18:13–9.
38. Mullur R, Liu YY, Brent GA. Thyroid hormone regulation of metabolism. Physiol Rev. 2014;94:355–82.
39. Rizos CV, Elisaf MS, Liberopoulos EN. Effects of thyroid dysfunction on lipid profile. Open Cardiovasc Med J. 2011;5:76–84.
40. dos Santos Teixeira PDF, Reuters VS, Ferreira MM, et al. Lipid profile in different degrees of hypothyroidism and effects of levothyroxine replacement in mild thyroid failure. Transl Res. 2008;151:224–31.
41. Liu P, Liu R, Chen X, et al. Can levothyroxine treatment reduce urinary albumin excretion rate in patients with early type 2 diabetic nephropathy and subclinical hypothyroidism? A randomized double-blind and placebo-controlled study. Curr Med Res Opin. 2015;31:2233–40.
42. Kowalska I, Borawski J, Nikołajuk A, et al. Insulin sensitivity, plasma adiponectin and sICAM-1 concentrations in patients with subclinical hypothyroidism: response to levothyroxine therapy. Endocrine. 2011;40:95–101.
43. Monzani F, Caraccio N, Kozàkowà M, et al. Effect of levothyroxine replacement on lipid profile and intima-media thickness in subclinical hypothyroidism: a double-blind, placebo-controlled study. J Clin Endocrinol Metab. 2004;89:2099–106.
44. Caraccio N, Ferrannini E, Monzani F. Lipoprotein profile in subclinical hypothyroidism: response to levothyroxine replacement, a randomized placebo-controlled study. J Clin Endocrinol Metab. 2002;87:1533–8.
45. Bruinstroop E, Dalan R, Cao Y, et al. Low-dose levothyroxine reduces intrahepatic lipid content in patients with type 2 diabetes mellitus and NAFLD. J Clin Endocrinol Metab. 2018;103:2698–706.
46. Bantle JP, Hunninghake DB, Frantz ID, Kuba K, Mariash CN, Oppenheimer JH. Comparison of effectiveness of thyrotropin-suppressive doses of D- and L-thyroxine in treatment of hypercholesterolemia. Am J Med. 1984;77:475–81.
47. Sanyal D, Raychaudhuri M. Hypothyroidism and obesity: an intriguing link. Indian J Endocrinol Metab. 2016;20:554–7.
48. Santini F, Marzullo P, Rotondi M, et al. Mechanisms in endocrinology: the crosstalk between thyroid gland and adipose tissue: signal integration in health and disease. Eur J Endocrinol. 2014;171:R137–52.
49. Bakiner O, Bozkirli E, Ersozlu Bozkirli ED, Ozsahin K. Correction of hypothyroidism seems to have no effect on body fat. Int J Endocrinol. 2013;2013:576794.
50. Mouradian M, Abourizk N. Diabetes mellitus and thyroid disease. Diabetes Care. 1983;6:512–20.
51. Nishi M. Diabetes mellitus and thyroid diseases. Diabetol Int. 2018;9:108–12.
52. Maxon HR, Kreines KW, Goldsmith RE, Knowles HC Jr. Long-term observations of glucose tolerance in thyrotoxic patients. Arch Intern Med. 1975;135:1477–80.
53. Ikeda T, Fujiyama K, Hoshino T, Takeuchi T, Mashiba H, Tominaga M. Oral and intravenous glucose-induced insulin secretion in hyperthyroid patients. Metabolism. 1990;39:633–7.
54. Komiya I, Yamada T, Sato A, Koizumi Y, Aoki T. Effects of antithyroid drug therapy on blood glucose, serum insulin, and insulin binding to red blood cells in hyperthyroid patients of different ages. Diabetes Care. 1985;8:161–8.
55. Taylor R, McCulloch AJ, Zeuzem S, Gray P, Clark F, Alberti KG. Insulin secretion, adipocyte insulin binding and insulin sensitivity in thyrotoxicosis. Acta Endocrinol (Copenh). 1985;109:96–103.

56. Jap TS, Ho LT, Won JG. Insulin secretion and sensitivity in hyperthyroidism. Horm Metab Res. 1989;21:261–6.
57. Dimitriadis GD, Raptis SA. Thyroid hormone excess and glucose intolerance. Exp Clin Endocrinol Diabetes. 2001;109(Suppl 2):S225–39.
58. Lambadiari V, Mitrou P, Maratou E, et al. Thyroid hormones are positively associated with insulin resistance early in the development of type 2 diabetes. Endocrine. 2011;39: 28–32.
59. Jing S, Xiaoying D, Ying X, et al. Different levels of thyroid hormones between impaired fasting glucose and impaired glucose tolerance: free T3 affects the prevalence of impaired fasting glucose and impaired glucose tolerance in opposite ways. Clin Endocrinol (Oxf). 2014;80:890–8.
60. Owecki M, El Ali Z, Nikisch E, Sowiński J. Serum insulin levels and the degree of thyroid dysfunction in hypothyroid women. Neuro Endocrinol Lett. 2008;29:137–40.
61. Maratou E, Hadjidakis DJ, Kollias A, et al. Studies of insulin resistance in patients with clinical and subclinical hypothyroidism. Eur J Endocrinol. 2009;160:785–90.
62. Kim SW, Jeon JH, Moon JS, et al. Low-normal free thyroxine levels in euthyroid male are associated with prediabetes. Diabetes Metab J. 2019;43:718–26.
63. Chaker L, Ligthart S, Korevaar TI, et al. Thyroid function and risk of type 2 diabetes: a population-based prospective cohort study. BMC Med. 2016;14:150.
64. Velija-Asimi Z, Karamehic J. The effects of treatment of subclinical hypothyroidism on metabolic control and hyperinsulinemia. Med Arh. 2007;61:20–1.
65. Stanicka S, Vondra K, Pelikanova T, Vlcek P, Hill M, Zamrazil V. Insulin sensitivity and counter-regulatory hormones in hypothyroidism and during thyroid hormone replacement therapy. Clin Chem Lab Med. 2005;43:715–20.
66. Roth J, Müller N, Kuniss N, Wolf G, Müller UA. Association between glycaemic control and the intake of thiazide diuretics, beta blockers and levothyroxine in people without diabetes. Exp Clin Endocrinol Diabetes. 2019; https://doi.org/10.1055/a-0919-4525.
67. Morini E, Catalano A, Lasco A, Morabito N, Benvenga S. L-thyroxine malabsorption due to calcium carbonate impairs blood pressure, total cholesterolemia, and fasting glycemia. Endocrine. 2019;64:284–92.
68. Heemstra KA, Smit JW, Eustatia-Rutten CF, et al. Glucose tolerance and lipid profile in long-term exogenous subclinical hyperthyroidism and the effects of restoration of euthyroidism, a randomised controlled trial. Clin Endocrinol (Oxf). 2006;65:737–44.
69. Hennessey JV, Scherger JE. Evaluating and treating the patient with hypothyroid disease. J Fam Pract. 2007;56(8 Suppl Hot Topics):S31–9.
70. Almeida C, Brasil MA, Costa AJ, et al. Subclinical hypothyroidism: psychiatric disorders and symptoms. Braz J Psychiatry. 2007;29:157–9.
71. Blum MR, Wijsman LW, Virgini VS, et al. Subclinical thyroid dysfunction and depressive symptoms among the elderly: a prospective cohort study. Neuroendocrinology. 2016;103:291–9.
72. Hong JW, Noh JH, Kim DJ. Association between subclinical thyroid dysfunction and depressive symptoms in the Korean adult population: the 2014 Korea National Health and Nutrition Examination Survey. PLoS One. 2018;13:e0202258.
73. Singh R, Tandon A, Gupta SK, Saroja K. Optimal levothyroxine replacement adequately improves symptoms of hypothyroidism; residual symptoms need further evaluation for other than hypothyroidism causation. Indian J Endocrinol Metab. 2017;21:830–5.
74. Brokhin M, Danzi S, Klein I. Assessment of the adequacy of thyroid hormone replacement therapy in hypothyroidism. Front Endocrinol (Lausanne). 2019;10:631.
75. Peterson SJ, McAninch EA, Bianco AC. Is a normal TSH synonymous with "euthyroidism" in levothyroxine monotherapy? J Clin Endocrinol Metab. 2016;101:4964–73.
76. Saravanan P, Chau WF, Roberts N, Vedhara K, Greenwood R, Dayan CM. Psychological well-being in patients on 'adequate' doses of l-thyroxine: results of a large, controlled community-based questionnaire study. Clin Endocrinol (Oxf). 2002;57:577–85.

77. Quinque EM, Villringer A, Kratzsch J, Karger S. Patient-reported outcomes in adequately treated hypothyroidism—insights from the German versions of ThyDQoL, ThySRQ and ThyTSQ. Health Qual Life Outcomes. 2013;11:68.
78. Peterson SJ, Cappola AR, Castro MR, et al. An online survey of hypothyroid patients demonstrates prominent dissatisfaction. Thyroid. 2018;28:707–21.
79. Najafi L, Malek M, Hadian A, Ebrahim Valojerdi A, Khamseh ME, Aghili R. Depressive symptoms in patients with subclinical hypothyroidism—the effect of treatment with levothyroxine: a double-blind randomized clinical trial. Endocr Res. 2015;40:121–6.
80. Romero-Gómez B, Guerrero-Alonso P, Carmona-Torres JM. Mood disorders in levothyroxine-treated hypothyroid women. Int J Environ Res Public Health. 2019;16:4776.
81. Talaei A, Rafee N, Rafei F, Chehrei A. TSH cut off point based on depression in hypothyroid patients. BMC Psychiatry. 2017;17:327.
82. Stewart AL, Greenfield S, Hays RD, et al. Functional status and well-being of patients with chronic conditions. Results from the medical outcomes study [published correction appears in JAMA 1989 Nov 10;262(18):2542]. JAMA. 1989;262:907–13.
83. Carta MG, Loviselli A, Hardoy MC, et al. The link between thyroid autoimmunity (antithyroid peroxidase autoantibodies) with anxiety and mood disorders in the community: a field of interest for public health in the future. BMC Psychiatry. 2004;4:25.
84. Groer MW, Vaughan JH. Positive thyroid peroxidase antibody titer is associated with dysphoric moods during pregnancy and postpartum. J Obstet Gynecol Neonatal Nurs. 2013;42:E26–32.
85. Panicker V, Saravanan P, Vaidya B, et al. Common variation in the DIO2 gene predicts baseline psychological well-being and response to combination thyroxine plus triiodothyronine therapy in hypothyroid patients. J Clin Endocrinol Metab. 2009;94:1623–9.
86. Kong WM, Sheikh MH, Lumb PJ, et al. A 6-month randomized trial of thyroxine treatment in women with mild subclinical hypothyroidism. Am J Med. 2002;112:348–54.
87. Ladenson PW. Psychological wellbeing in patients. Clin Endocrinol (Oxf). 2002;57:575–6.
88. Pollock MA, Sturrock A, Marshall K, et al. Thyroxine treatment in patients with symptoms of hypothyroidism but thyroid function tests within the reference range: randomised double blind placebo controlled crossover trial. BMJ. 2001;323:891–5.
89. Stamm TJ, Lewitzka U, Sauer C, et al. Supraphysiologic doses of levothyroxine as adjunctive therapy in bipolar depression: a randomized, double-blind, placebo-controlled study. J Clin Psychiatry. 2014;75:162–8.
90. Bauer M, Berman S, Stamm T, et al. Levothyroxine effects on depressive symptoms and limbic glucose metabolism in bipolar disorder: a randomized, placebo-controlled positron emission tomography study. Mol Psychiatry. 2016;21:229–36.
91. Bauer M, London ED, Rasgon N, et al. Supraphysiological doses of levothyroxine alter regional cerebral metabolism and improve mood in bipolar depression. Mol Psychiatry. 2005;10:456–69.
92. Samuels MH, Kolobova I, Smeraglio A, Peters D, Janowsky JS, Schuff KG. The effects of levothyroxine replacement or suppressive therapy on health status, mood, and cognition. J Clin Endocrinol Metab. 2014;99:843–51.
93. Cathébras PJ, Robbins JM, Kirmayer LJ, Hayton BC. Fatigue in primary care: prevalence, psychiatric comorbidity, illness behavior, and outcome. J Gen Intern Med. 1992;7:276–86.
94. Stadje R, Dornieden K, Baum E, et al. The differential diagnosis of tiredness: a systematic review. BMC Fam Pract. 2016;17:147.
95. Canaris GJ, Steiner JF, Ridgway EC. Do traditional symptoms of hypothyroidism correlate with biochemical disease? J Gen Intern Med. 1997;12:544–50.
96. Canaris GJ, Manowitz NR, Mayor G, Ridgway EC. The Colorado thyroid disease prevalence study. Arch Intern Med. 2000;160:526–34.
97. Carlé A, Pedersen IB, Knudsen N, et al. Hypothyroid symptoms fail to predict thyroid insufficiency in old people: a population-based case-control study. Am J Med. 2016;129:1082–92.

98. Wouters H. Abstract OR34-1 and oral presentation at: the endocrine society annual meeting, Chicago, USA, 17–20 Mar 2018.
99. Massolt ET, van der Windt M, Korevaar TI, et al. Thyroid hormone and its metabolites in relation to quality of life in patients treated for differentiated thyroid cancer. Clin Endocrinol (Oxf). 2016;85:781–8.
100. Krysiak R, Okopien B. The effect of levothyroxine and selenomethionine on lymphocyte and monocyte cytokine release in women with Hashimoto's thyroiditis. J Clin Endocrinol Metab. 2011;96:2206–15.
101. Bilgir O, Bilgir F, Calan M, Calan OG, Yuksel A. Comparison of pre- and post-levothyroxine high-sensitivity c-reactive protein and fetuin-a levels in subclinical hypothyroidism. Clinics (Sao Paulo). 2015;70:97–101.
102. Gullo S, Sav H, Kamel N. Effects of levothyroxine treatment on biochemical and hemostasis parameters in patients with hypothyroidism. Eur J Endocrinol. 2005;152:355–61.
103. Elbers LPB, Fliers E, Cannegieter SC. The influence of thyroid function on the coagulation system and its clinical consequences. J Thromb Haemost. 2018;16:634–45.
104. Manfredi E, van Zaane B, Gerdes VE, Brandjes DP, Squizzato A. Hypothyroidism and acquired von Willebrand's syndrome: a systematic review. Haemophilia. 2008;14:423–33.
105. Debeij J, van Zaane B, Dekkers OM, et al. High levels of procoagulant factors mediate the association between free thyroxine and the risk of venous thrombosis: the MEGA study. J Thromb Haemost. 2014;12:839–46.
106. van Zaane B, Squizzato A, Huijgen R, et al. Increasing levels of free thyroxine as a risk factor for a first venous thrombosis: a case-control study. Blood. 2010;115:4344–9.
107. Lupoli R, Di Minno MN, Tortora A, et al. Primary and secondary hemostasis in patients with subclinical hypothyroidism: effect of levothyroxine treatment. J Clin Endocrinol Metab. 2015;100:2659–65.
108. Guldiken S, Demir M, Turgut B, Altun BU, Arikan E, Kara M. Global fibrinolytic capacity in patients with subclinical hypothyroidism. Endocr J. 2005;52:363–7.
109. Akinci B, Comlekci A, Ali Ozcan M, et al. Elevated thrombin activatable fibrinolysis inhibitor (TAFI) antigen levels in overt and subclinical hypothyroid patients were reduced by levothyroxine replacement. Endocr J. 2007;54:45–52.
110. Chadarevian R, Jublanc C, Bruckert E, et al. Effect of levothyroxine replacement therapy on coagulation and fibrinolysis in severe hypothyroidism. J Endocrinol Investig. 2005;28:398–404.
111. Desideri G, Bocale R, D'Amore A, et al. Replacement therapy with levothyroxine modulates platelet activation in recent-onset post-thyroidectomy subclinical hypothyroidism. Nutr Metab Cardiovasc Dis. 2017;27:896–901.
112. Lippi G, Salvagno GL, Rugolotto S, et al. Routine coagulation tests in newborn and young infants. J Thromb Thrombolysis. 2007;24:153–5.
113. Li Y, Chen H, Tan J, Wang X, Liang H, Sun X. Impaired release of tissue plasminogen activator from the endothelium in Graves' disease—indicator of endothelial dysfunction and reduced fibrinolytic capacity. Eur J Clin Investig. 1998;28:1050–4.
114. Liu L, Wang X, Lin Z, Wu H. Elevated plasma levels of VWF: Ag in hyperthyroidism are mediated through beta-adrenergic receptors. Endocr Res. 1993;19:123–33.
115. Myrup B, Bregengård C, Faber J. Primary haemostasis in thyroid disease. J Intern Med. 1995;238:59–63.
116. Sheu JJ, Kang JH, Lin HC, Lin HC. Hyperthyroidism and risk of ischemic stroke in young adults: a 5-year follow-up study. Stroke. 2010;41:961–6.
117. Elbers LP, Moran C, Gerdes VE, et al. The hypercoagulable state in hyperthyroidism is mediated via the thyroid hormone β receptor pathway. Eur J Endocrinol. 2016; https://doi.org/10.1530/EJE-15-1249.
118. Akinci B, Demir T, Comlekci A, et al. Effect of levothyroxine suppression therapy on plasma thrombin activatable fibrinolysis inhibitor antigen levels in benign thyroid nodules. Med Princ Pract. 2011;20:23–8.

119. Demir T, Akinci B, Comlekci A, et al. Levothyroxine (LT4) suppression treatment for benign thyroid nodules alters coagulation. Clin Endocrinol (Oxf). 2009;71:446–50.
120. Hooper JM, Stuijver DJ, Orme SM, et al. Thyroid dysfunction and fibrin network structure: a mechanism for increased thrombotic risk in hyperthyroid individuals. J Clin Endocrinol Metab. 2012;97:1463–73.
121. Van Zaane B, Squizzato A, Debeij J, et al. Alterations in coagulation and fibrinolysis after levothyroxine exposure in healthy volunteers: a controlled randomized crossover study. J Thromb Haemost. 2011;9:1816–24.
122. Kreisman SH, Hennessey JV. Consistent reversible elevations of serum creatinine levels in severe hypothyroidism. Arch Intern Med. 1999;159:79–82.
123. Shin DH, Lee MJ, Kim SJ, et al. Preservation of renal function by thyroid hormone replacement therapy in chronic kidney disease patients with subclinical hypothyroidism. J Clin Endocrinol Metab. 2012;97:2732–40.
124. Sawka AM, Carty SE, Haugen BR, et al. American Thyroid Association guidelines and statements: past, present, and future. Thyroid. 2018;28:692–706.
125. Jonklaas J, Bianco AC, Bauer AJ, et al. Guidelines for the treatment of hypothyroidism: prepared by the American Thyroid Association Task Force on Thyroid Hormone Replacement. Thyroid. 2014;24:1670–751.
126. Thyroid disease: assessment and management. NICE guideline [NG145]. Nov 2019. Available at https://www.nice.org.uk/guidance/ng145/chapter/Recommendations. Accessed Jul 2020.
127. Stott DJ, Rodondi N, Kearney PM, et al. Thyroid hormone therapy for older adults with subclinical hypothyroidism. N Engl J Med. 2017;376:2534–44.
128. Surks MI, Hollowell JG. Age-specific distribution of serum thyrotropin and antithyroid antibodies in the US population: implications for the prevalence of subclinical hypothyroidism. J Clin Endocrinol Metab. 2007;92:4575–82.
129. Feller M, Snel M, Moutzouri E, et al. Association of thyroid hormone therapy with quality of life and thyroid-related symptoms in patients with subclinical hypothyroidism: a systematic review and meta-analysis. JAMA. 2018;320:1349–59.
130. Pearce SH, Brabant G, Duntas LH, et al. 2013 ETA guideline: management of subclinical hypothyroidism. Eur Thyroid J. 2013;2:215–28.
131. Bekkering GE, Agoritsas T, Lytvyn L, et al. Thyroid hormones treatment for subclinical hypothyroidism: a clinical practice guideline. BMJ. 2019;365:l2006.
132. Biondi B, Cappola AR, Cooper DS. Subclinical hypothyroidism: a review. JAMA. 2019;322:153–60.
133. Somwaru LL, Rariy CM, Arnold AM, Cappola AR. The natural history of subclinical hypothyroidism in the elderly: the cardiovascular health study. J Clin Endocrinol Metab. 2012;97:1962–9.
134. Paragliola RM, Corsello A, Concolino P, et al. Iodothyronine deiodinases and reduced sensitivity to thyroid hormones. Front Biosci (Landmark Ed). 2020;25:201–28.
135. Hennessey JV, Espaillat R. Current evidence for the treatment of hypothyroidism with levothyroxine/levotriiodothyronine combination therapy versus levothyroxine monotherapy. Int J Clin Pract. 2018;72:e13062.
136. Hennessey JV. Historical and current perspective in the use of thyroid extracts for the treatment of hypothyroidism. Endocr Pract. 2015;21:1161–70.
137. Wiersinga WM, Duntas L, Fadeyev V, Nygaard B, Vanderpump MP. 2012 ETA guidelines: the use of L-T4 + L-T3 in the treatment of hypothyroidism. Eur Thyroid J. 2012;1:55–71.
138. Jonklaas J, Tefera E, Shara N. Physician choice of hypothyroidism therapy: influence of patient characteristics. Thyroid. 2018;28:1416–24.
139. DiStefano J 3rd, Jonklaas J. Predicting optimal combination LT4 + LT3 therapy for hypothyroidism based on residual thyroid function. Front Endocrinol (Lausanne). 2019;10:746.

140. Okosieme O, Gilbert J, Abraham P, et al. Management of primary hypothyroidism: statement by the British Thyroid Association Executive Committee. Clin Endocrinol (Oxf). 2016;84:799–808.
141. Jørgensen P, Langhammer A, Krokstad S, Forsmo S. Diagnostic labelling influences self-rated health. A prospective cohort study: the HUNT Study, Norway. Fam Pract. 2015;32:492–9.
142. Bould H, Panicker V, Kessler D, et al. Investigation of thyroid dysfunction is more likely in patients with high psychological morbidity. Fam Pract. 2012;29:163–7.
143. Walsh JP, Ward LC, Burke V, et al. Small changes in thyroxine dosage do not produce measurable changes in hypothyroid symptoms, well-being, or quality of life: results of a double-blind, randomized clinical trial. J Clin Endocrinol Metab. 2006;91:2624–30.
144. Samuels MH, Kolobova I, Niederhausen M, Janowsky JS, Schuff KG. Effects of altering levothyroxine (L-T4) doses on quality of life, mood, and cognition in L-T4 treated subjects. J Clin Endocrinol Metab. 2018;103:1997–2008.

Levothyroxine in Pregnancy

Kris Gustave Poppe

Thyroid hormone homeostasis changes markedly during pregnancy, and first trimester-specific reference ranges for thyrotropin (thyroid-stimulating hormone, TSH) are needed to diagnose hypothyroidism. Treatment consists in levothyroxine (LT4) in this setting (triiodothyronine or desiccated thyroid preparations have no role here). Severe hypothyroidism is associated with infertility, and levels of TSH above 4.0 IU/mL signal an increased risk of adverse pregnancy outcomes. All pregnant women (and women planning a pregnancy) with overt hypothyroidism must be managed effectively with oral LT4. Thyroid autoimmunity increases the risk of adverse pregnancy outcomes and is associated with certain causes of infertility. Current European and US guidelines recommend a role for patients with subclinical hypothyroidism and thyroid autoimmunity, not least to guard against progression to overt hypothyroidism during the pregnancy. Women with hypothyroidism undergoing assisted reproduction technology to become pregnant appear to be strong candidates for LT4-based therapy.

1 Introduction

About 1% of pregnant women have overt hypothyroidism (OH) and about 10% have subclinical hypothyroidism (SCH) during pregnancy [1]. This chapter will address the issue of hypothyroidism in women who are pregnant, planning a pregnancy (with or without assisted reproductive technology [ART]), or who

K. G. Poppe (✉)
Endocrine Unit, Centre Hospitalier Universitaire Saint Pierre, Brussels, Belgium

Université Libre de Bruxelles (ULB), Brussels, Belgium
e-mail: kris_POPPE@stpierre-bru.be

are in the immediate postpartum period. Topics to be discussed will include the impact of pregnancy on the management of hypothyroidism, the effects of hypothyroidism and its management with levothyroxine (LT4) on maternal and neonatal outcomes, and the current status of guidelines for the management of these patients.

2   Changes in Thyroid Function During Pregnancy

A number of changes take place due to the presence of the placenta and the foetus [2, 3]. During the first trimester of pregnancy, the foetus is dependent on thyroid hormones of the mother, and at the same time, placental deiodinase type 3 protects it against an excess, by degrading them. Other changes necessitating an increased production of thyroid hormones in the mother are the increased urinary iodine clearance, and thyroxine-binding globulin (TBG) levels due to the higher oestradiol concentrations. This latter phenomenon takes place earlier and is more accentuated if an ovarian hyperstimulation (OS) takes place for a pregnancy conceived using ART. On the other hand, increasing human chorionic gonadotrophin stimulates maternal thyroid to augment thyroid hormone production. Therefore, the thyrotropin level decreases during the first trimester, which partially reverses as the pregnancy progresses [2, 3].

All these changes can lead to the development of (subclinical) hypothyroidism during pregnancy especially where women have severe iodine deficiency, thyroid autoimmunity (TAI), or do not take enough LT4 after thyroid surgery.

Pregnancy markedly increases the dose of LT4 required to control TSH, with changes in LT4 requirement varying according to the aetiology of the hypothyroid state and thyroid status before pregnancy [2–5]. For example, longitudinal studies in pregnant women with hypothyroidism showed that the dose of LT4 needed to control TSH adequately (<2.5 mIU/L) increased by about half during the first trimester and remained relatively stable for the remainder of the pregnancy [6, 7]. This is not a universal finding during pregnancy, however, and a minority of patients in the larger of these studies required no increase in the LT4 dose, and a few even required a dose decrease [6]. Another study, in 19 women, showed that the LT4 dose increased by 47% in the first trimester, and then remained at this level throughout the pregnancy. Current guidelines (see below) recommend an immediate increase in the dose of LT4 when pregnancy is discovered. Postpartum, thyroid function, and LT4 requirements return to pre-pregnancy levels for most patients though some continue to require a higher dose than that received before the pregnancy [6, 8]. In women pregnant after ART, the increase in the LT4 dose is higher and takes place earlier in pregnancy [8]. The presence of TAI is the sole condition that predicts the fact that LT4 will have to be increased during pregnancy, both in spontaneous and assisted pregnancies [6, 9].

3 Maternal and Foetal Outcomes in Women with Hypothyroidism

3.1 Effects of Hypothyroidism on Fertility and Preterm Delivery

Severe overt hypothyroidism decreases fertility through its actions on the production of sex hormone-binding globulin (decreased) and prolactin (increased), and via a direct impact on the ovaries [10]. In a meta-analysis of 19 cohort studies (involving a total of 47,045 pregnancies), SCH was associated with an increased risk of preterm delivery, with an odds ratio (OR) 1.04 (95%CI, 1.00–1.09) for each increase in TSH of one standard deviation [11]. The presence of antibodies to thyroid peroxidase also increased the risk of preterm delivery in this study (OR 1.33; 95%CI, 1.15–1.56). In women with iodine deficiency (urinary iodine <100 µg/L) TSH ≥4.0 mIU/L was associated with a 2.5-fold ($p = 0.024$) increased risk of preterm delivery, compared with lower TSH levels, in the population-based Tehran Thyroid and Pregnancy Study [12]. In another study, inadequately controlled hypothyroidism was associated with an increased risk of miscarriage, especially where TSH level exceeded 4.5 mIU/L [13].

3.2 LT4 Treatment and Pregnancy Outcomes: Importance of Thyroid Autoimmunity

A placebo- (or no treatment-) controlled evaluation of LT4 in pregnant women with overt hypothyroidism would be unethical, given the known association of markedly elevated TSH with miscarriage [14]. Overt hypothyroidism should always be treated with LT4 during pregnancy, as in other settings [14].

Most evidence relating to the effects of LT4 on pregnancy outcomes has come from clinical studies in women with SCH. A randomised trial in 64 infertile women with SCH undergoing in vitro fertilisation (IVF) and intracellular sperm injection (ICSI) found a higher embryo implantation rate and live birth rate, associated with a lower miscarriage rate, in subjects randomised to LT4 vs. no LT4 [15]. The study population was not selected for the presence of TAI *per se* though higher anti-TPO and anti-Tg levels predicted a higher risk of miscarriage in the control group. The potential influence of TAI on pregnancy outcomes in LT4-treated women undergoing ICSI is discussed in more detail later in this chapter.

A meta-analysis of 13 randomised and observational studies included more than 11,000 women with SCH [16]. Treatment vs. no treatment with LT4 in this analysis affected different pregnancy outcomes in different ways, with fewer lost pregnancies (OR 0.78; 95% CI 0.66–0.94) and more live birth rates (OR 2.72; 95% CI 1.44–5.11), but a higher chance of premature labour (OR 1.82; 95% CI 1.14–2.91).

Increasing the dose of LT4 for women with TSH >2.5 mIU/L in the first trimester was also associated with a ~15-fold reduction in the frequency of preterm birth, compared with pregnant women whose LT4 dose remained stable, according to a retrospective analysis [17]. However, there appeared to be no upper limit for TSH in this study, and the median TSH level before the LT4 dose increase was 5.0 mIU/L.

The appearance of TAI is also strongly associated with certain causes of infertility, in particular polycystic ovary syndrome and idiopathic infertility [10]. Numerous studies have addressed the impact of TAI on pregnancy outcomes, following the initial finding of a two-fold increase in the risk of miscarriage associated with anti-TPO-Ab and/or anti-Tg-Ab three decades ago [18]. Meta-analyses have confirmed these initial findings consistently, with odds for miscarriage ratios of 2.31 (cohort studies in women with vs. without TAI) [19], 2.55 (case-control studies from the same meta-analysis) [19], 2.8 (women with vs. without SCH or TPO-Ab who had undergone ART [20], 3.9 (cohort studies of euthyroid women with vs. without TAI) [21], 1.8 (case-control studies from the same meta-analysis), 21 and 1.44 (women with vs. without TAI undergoing ART) [22]. Furthermore, a recent (retrospective) analysis demonstrated a 17-fold increase in the requirement for neonatal intensive care treatment associated with TAI [23].

Two recent meta-analyses in both spontaneous and assisted pregnancies have appeared recently, from the same group published one year apart (2018–2019), finding that treatment with LT4 was associated with less pregnancy loss and fewer preterm births in women with SCH and TAI [24, 25]. A further meta-analysis (14 randomised or observational trials) focussed on women with SCH and/or TAI and found that LT4 vs. placebo or no treatment was associated with reduced risk of a range of adverse outcomes (higher fertilisation and delivery rates, lower rates of miscarriages, gestational diabetes, and gestational hypertension, preterm deliveries, and low birth weights) [26].

A prospective study compared the effects of LT4 vs. no treatment on pregnancy outcomes in 131 patients with SCH (TSH could be as high as 10 mIU/L) and TPO-Ab [27]. LT4 treatment was associated with fewer preterm deliveries vs. no treatment or a euthyroid, TPO-Ab–control group. Finally, a report from the Tehran Thyroid and Pregnancy Study described randomisation of 366 pregnant women with SCH (TSH cut-off 2.5 mIU/L), but no TPO-Ab, to LT4 or no treatment [28]. LT4 did not affect the risk of adverse pregnancy outcomes. Interestingly, there was a significant reduction for LT4 vs. no treatment for preterm delivery for patients with TSH >4.0 IU/L.

Accordingly, the results of clinical studies in women with SCH have been conflicting, with regard to the effects of LT4 on pregnancy outcomes. This might be due to the use of TSH >2.5 mIU/L as cut-off to define SCH during the period 2005–2016. Most studies defining SCH as a TSH >4.0 mIU/L or above the upper limit of the reference range for non-pregnant women show beneficial effects of LT4 on pregnancy outcomes.

3.3 LT4 Treatment of Euthyroid Women with Thyroid Autoimmunity

Two randomised trials have been conducted in euthyroid women with TAI. The Thyroid Antibodies and Levothyroxine study (TABLET) randomised 952 women with TPO-Ab and a history of miscarriage or infertility to treatment with LT4 50 µg or placebo from before conception to the end of the pregnancy. There were no differences between groups in the live birth rate (primary outcome) or the number of miscarriages [29]. In an earlier (2006), smaller, randomised trial in women with TPO-Ab not selected for the presence of thyroid dysfunction, treatment with LT4 was associated with a lower miscarriage rate, compared with no LT4 treatment [30].

Other evidence in this area is from meta-analyses and observational studies. One meta-analyses demonstrated no marked effect of LT4 supplementation on pregnancy outcomes in euthyroid women with TAI [31]. Administration of LT4 of women with loss of at least two prior pregnancies and TSH 2.5–4.0 mIU/L did not influence the success of a subsequent pregnancy significantly, and TPO antibody status did not modify this finding, in an observational study [32]. On the contrary, in a recent large cohort of women with unexplained recurrent pregnancy loss, TPO-Ab positivity was predictive of a reduced live birth rate, and furthermore, LT4 improved odds of live birth [33]. More randomised controlled trials are needed to resolve this issue.

An additional case-control study found no dose-related effect of LT4 treatment on pregnancy outcomes, compared with an untreated control group, in euthyroid women without TAI, despite significant changes in placental function markers [34]. These data support the current recommendation that euthyroid women without TAI, including those with high-normal TSH levels, may not require intervention with LT4 treatment (see below). A single-centre, cross-sectional analysis of 1321 women without thyroid disease showed that variation of the TSH level within normal range for non-pregnant women did not increase the risk of adverse pregnancy outcomes, including gestational diabetes, pre-eclampsia, postpartum haemorrhage, intra-uterine growth retardation, or low birth weight [35].

3.4 Thyroid Autoimmunity and Pregnancy Outcomes in Women Receiving Assisted Reproduction Technologies (ART)

Thyroid autoimmunity is common among women seeking treatment for infertility: one study of detected thyroid autoantibodies in 16% of an unselected cohort women attending specialist care for this reason [36]. The majority (12%) had anti-TPO-Ab ± anti-thyroglobulin antibodies (anti-Tg-Ab), and 5% had only anti-Tg-Ab. However, most studies in this area have been based on detection of anti-TPO-Ab, which is more often measured routinely [14].

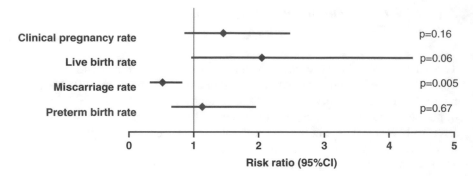

Fig. 1 Effects of LT4 on pregnancy outcomes from a meta-analysis of studies in women with subclinical hypothyroidism undergoing assisted reproduction. Risk ratios >1 signify higher likelihood of event in the levothyroxine vs. control group; *p* values are for overall effect. (Drawn from data presented in Ref. [24])

Observations of increased miscarriage rates associated with TAI (see above) have prompted evaluations of LT4 in euthyroid women with anti-thyroid antibodies receiving ART. Another study found that randomisation of such a population to LT4 (25 μg [TSH <2.5 mIU/L] or 50 μg [TSH ≥2.5 mIU/L]) vs. placebo had no significant effect on miscarriage rates (primary outcome) or on clinical pregnancy rates or live birth rates (secondary outcomes) [37]. An accompanying editorial welcomed the study, but noted its relatively low miscarriage rate, compared with other, similar populations, and the relatively low proportion of pregnancies achieved using ICSI about half [38]. Moreover, previous neutral evaluations of LT4 in similar populations were underpowered and/or non-randomised [30, 39].

A recent meta-analysis of 765 pregnancies achieved using ICSI showed that the rate of miscarriage in these women was unaffected by TAI [40]. This is an opposite result compared with previous meta-analyses on the impact of TAI on pregnancy outcomes, as described above. More studies are needed to find out whether this is due to the use of ICSI or because studies were included that used a cut-off for TSH of 3.0 mIU/L (or lower) to define SCH. An argument in favour of the latter hypothesis is a meta-analysis from Velkeniers et al. (published in 2013), in which LT4 treatment vs. no additional treatment decreased the miscarriage rate and increased the live birth rate in women with SCH (defined by TSH levels >4.0 mIU/L) achieving pregnancy through ART (Fig. 1) [20]. However, no beneficial impact of LT4 was noted in women with TAI undergoing ART in a more recent meta-analysis in which SCH was defined in the majority of included studies by TSH <4.0 mIU/L [24].

ICSI and LT4 may work together to improve outcomes especially when ICSI is used to assist conception: ICSI may bypass inhibitory effects of thyroid antibodies in the follicular fluid that surrounds the ovum, while LT4 preserves a more normal hypothalamic-pituitary-thyroid axis after implantation [38].

A cross-sectional study in 279 women undergoing ART found that either TSH above vs. below 2.5 mIU/L in women without TAI, or the presence vs. absence of TPO-Ab, did not affect the quality of oocytes retrieved, the fertilisation rate or the quality of the subsequent embryos [41]. Further studies are needed, to investigate whether LT4 could improve the ovarian reserve or in vitro outcomes of an ART procedure.

3.5 Effects on Offspring

Cognitive outcomes in children born to mothers with hypothyroidism is also an active area of research. Low T4 levels in mothers have been associated significantly with delayed cognitive development in their children in some [42, 43] but not all [44] studies. A meta-analysis, of three randomised trials conducted in women diagnosed with SCH during pregnancy, found no effect of LT4 treatment on children's neuropsychological outcomes [45]. Treatment of hypothyroid mothers in the second trimester did not improve neurocognitive outcomes in the offspring [46]. A follow-up study to the Tehran Thyroid and Pregnancy Study will evaluate the neurocognitive development of 3-year old children born to mothers with mild hypothyroidism (without TAI) [47].

4 Summary of Current Major Guidelines

4.1 Guidelines Considered Here

Guidelines from Europe (on subclinical hypothyroidism) [48] and the USA (a broad guideline considering most aspects of hypothyroidism [14]) will be considered here, as examples of major guidelines with international reach. Many other guidelines are available for other regions: it is beyond the scope of this chapter to review them all, and chapter, "Practical Application of Levothyroxine-Based Therapy" of this book lists a number of them.

4.2 Overt Hypothyroidism During Pregnancy and Postpartum

The American Thyroid Association (ATA) published a major guideline on the management of thyroid disease in 2017 [14]. This comprehensive guidance covered all aspects of thyroid dysfunction and stated 109 clinical questions that were answered by 111 recommendations. Table 1 provides an overview of these recommendations, grouped under convenient subheadings, and a brief description of the main points with regard to LT4 therapy follows.

Briefly, diagnosis of maternal hypothyroidism should be conducted using trimester-specific reference ranges for TSH, ideally specific to a particular assay used, and defined in local, healthy, euthyroid, pregnant women without TPO-Abs. Depending on these factors, serum TSH values defining SCH during the first trimester will be >3.5–4.5 mIU/L. Measurement of TSH is recommended regularly for women at risk of thyroid disease (e.g. due to TAI or SCH). General screening for elevated TSH is not supported for women at low risk for thyroid disease, with the exception of women undergoing ART.

Table 1 Overview of principal recommendations from the American Thyroid Association regarding the management of hypothyroidism during pregnancy

Measure TSH	• In women under care for infertility • At start of pregnancy, and every 4 weeks through mid-pregnancy and at least once near 30 weeks gestation in women with thyroid Abs • *Measure TSH 2 weeks after controlled ovarian stimulation during ART, as this renders test results difficult to interpret (repeat at 2–4 weeks if TSH is high)* • *No support for universal screening for abnormal TSH in women without risk factors for thyroid disease (except for those planning ART)*
Diagnosis	• Maternal hypothyroidism = TSH > upper limit of trimester-specific reference range • Use assay-specific reference ranges (if possible locally derived from healthy, I-replete, TPO-Ab—pregnant women without thyroid illness) • Use an upper reference limit of ~4 mIU/L where such reference ranges are not available • TT4 measurement is a suitable alternative to FT4 later in pregnancy
Iodine and other supplements	• Use median urinary iodine concentrations, not spot or 24 h measurements to determine iodine status in an individual • Pregnant women need ~250 μg iodine/day, usually via a potassium iodide supplement (*an annual dose of iodised oil is a temporary solution for some I-depleted low-resource areas*) • No need for iodine supplementation if a woman is taking LT4 • Avoid excessive iodine exposure during pregnancy (except pre-surgery for Graves' disease) due to concerns about causing hypothyroidism in the foetus • Breastfeeding women should take iodine supplementation (similar to above; all breastfeeding women should ingest a ~250 μg iodine/day)
Use of LT4 during pregnancy	• Counsel hypothyroid women of an increased requirement for LT4 during pregnancy: if pregnancy occurs, they should increase their LT4 dose by about 20–30% and contact/see their physician promptly • Use oral LT4 for all women with overt hypothyroidism who are planning pregnancy, or during pregnancy; *aim for lower half of trimester-specific reference range for TSH (or TSH <2.5 mIU/L)* • There is insufficient evidence for routine use of LT4 for women with subclinical hypothyroidism without thyroid autoimmunity who are trying to become pregnant—but, LT4 may be considered as it may prevent progression to overt hypothyroidism • Do not use LT4 + T3 or desiccated thyroid preparations • *Consider LT4 for TPO-Ab + women with prior recurrent idiopathic pregnancy loss* • *Do not routinely treat isolated hypothyroxinaemia (low FT4 with normal TSH)* • Maintain TSH at the preconception level for pregnant women with thyroid cancer

Table 1 (continued)

Postpartum	• Reduce LT4 dose to the preconception level after delivery, check TSH ~6 w postpartum (some women do not need LT4 postpartum, especially where the dose was <50 µg)
	• Check thyroid status for otherwise unexplained lack of milk production
	• Treat hypothyroidism irrespective of severity in women seeking to breastfeed
	• TSH measurement to follow course of postpartum thyroiditis (PPT; including annually in women with prior PPT) and *consider LT4 for the hypothyroid phase (discontinue LT4 by ~12 months in the absence of new pregnancy)*
	• Do not use LT4 to prevent PPT in euthyroid, Ab+ pregnant women

Selected recommendations relating to the management of overt hypothyroidism are summarised here; these have been paraphrased, and in some cases aggregated, for brevity: see the full guideline. "Weak" recommendations are shown in italics; others are "Strong". Compiled from information presented in Ref. [14]

Oral LT4 is the mainstay of treatment of overt hypothyroidism during or leading up to a pregnancy, as for other populations with hypothyroidism. The guideline strongly recommends against the use of LT4 + LT3 combinations, or the use of desiccated thyroid preparations for treatment, a practice, which continues in spite of a lack of evidence of benefit, an evidence for harm, during pregnancy [49]. In general, targeting the lower half of the TSH reference range is supported for women with hypothyroidism who are, or who are planning to become pregnant. Women should be educated on the likelihood of a steep rise in LT4 requirement during pregnancy and should be ready to increase their LT4 dose on discovering a pregnancy *before* seeking prompt advice from their healthcare team. In daily practice, this could be implemented by adding two LT4 tablets a week at confirmation of the pregnancy [50]. LT4 requirements decrease postpartum, sometimes to zero, especially where the maintenance dose during pregnancy was low (<50 µg).

LT4 treatment may be considered also for the management of the hypothyroid phase of postpartum thyroiditis (PPT), which classically follows a transient hyperthyroid phase and occurs from 3 to 12 months postpartum. Indications to treat are women with symptomatic hypothyroidism and/or TSH values >10 mIU/L. In 10–20% of the cases, the hypothyroidism can be permanent, depending on pre-existing thyroid dysfunction (elevation of TSH and TPO-Ab levels). In most women, the duration of LT4 therapy, once initiated, is uncertain. It is reasonable to start weaning patients off treatment after 6–12 months of treatment, in the absence of a new pregnancy or decision to breastfeed [14].

It is important to note that LT4 treatment does not prevent PPT. Finally, oral LT4 may be considered for hypothyroid women who lack milk production, once other possible causes have been excluded. Breastfeeding *per se* is not a contraindication to LT4 treatment.

The ATA guidance considered that there was insufficient evidence to support the use of LT4 with the intention of preventing pregnancy loss, for euthyroid women with TAI, a position that is likely to be strengthened by the recent results of the TABLET study, described above. However, a weak recommendation supports the administration of a low dose of LT4 (typically starting at 25–50 µg) to women with TAI undergoing ART, given the possibility of benefit vs. minimal risk. One more indication (not as yet in the ATA guidance) could be women with recurrent idio-pathic miscarriage and TAI (see above) [33].

A guideline on the management of SCH from the European Thyroid Association (ETA), published in 2014 [48], contains some recommendations on the manage-ment of overt hypothyroidism. These are in general compatible with the ATA guide-line. In particular, this guideline agreed with the later ATA guidance on:

- The use of LT4, rather than combination therapy or desiccated thyroid products.
- The principle of managing TSH to the lower half of its trimester-specific refer-ence range.
- The return to the preconception dose of LT4 postpartum.

The ETA guideline differs from the ATA guideline in providing low-strength support for the use of LT4 for managing isolated hypothyroxinaemia in the first trimester, on the basis of an association of this condition with neuropsychological impairment on the neonate.

Other guidance summarised in Table 1 concerns the maintenance of adequate iodine intake. This is included for completeness and will not be discussed further here. Similar recommendations are provided in the ETA guideline for SCH (see the full guideline for details) [48].

4.3   Subclinical Hypothyroidism During Pregnancy and Postpartum

The principal sources of guidance for the management of SCH are from the 2014 guideline from the ETA [48] and the 2017 ATA guideline, described above for the management of overt hypothyroidism [14].

The ETA guideline notes the likely association between SCH and a range of adverse pregnancy outcomes (pregnancy loss, gestational diabetes, gestational hypertension, pre-eclampsia, and preterm delivery), while acknowledging the con-flicting results of some of these studies (see above). Accordingly, the ETA guideline supports treating women diagnosed with SCH before and during pregnancy with oral LT4 (Table 2). Both the ETA and ATA guidelines provide stronger recommen-dations on the use of oral LT4 treatment for women who are TPO-Ab+ (Table 2). The ATA guideline further supports LT4 treatment of women with SCH who are receiving ART or are breastfeeding (Table 2).

No recommendation was provided on screening for SCH was made by the ETA, due to a lack of evidence, consistent with the views of the ATA, discussed above. The authorship was split on this issue, however, with some authors noting that such an approach would avoid the danger of pregnancies being exposed to undiagnosed overt hypothyroidism. This uncertainty has been reflected in clinical practice, where survey evidence identified marked differences within Europe with respect to screen-ing for hypothyroidism in pregnancy [51]. The ATA guideline noted that prevention of progression to overt hypothyroidism is an advantage of detecting SCH early in the pregnancy.

Table 2 Comparison of European and US guideline recommendations on the use of LT4 to manage subclinical hypothyroidism in pregnant women, or women planning a pregnancy

Patients	ETA recommendations (2014)	ATA recommendations (2017)
TPO-Ab+	**Recommends use of oral LT4** to maintain TSH <2.5 mIU/L in women planning pregnancy, especially those who are TPO-Ab+ (level 2 recommendation) **Recommends use of oral LT4** for women with newly diagnosed subclinical hypothyroidism to control TSH to within its trimester-specific reference range (no recommendation level provided)	**Recommends use of oral LT4** where TSH is above the trimester-specific reference range (strong recommendation) **Consider use of oral LT4** where TSH is between 2.5 mIU/L and the top of the trimester-specific reference range (weak recommendation)
TPO-Ab−	**Recommends use of oral LT4 to maintain TSH <2.5 mIU/L for women with subclinical hypothyroidism** (level 2 recommendation) **Stop LT4 after pregnancy** if TSH <5 mIU/L (level 2 recommendation)	**Recommends use of oral LT4** where TSH is >10 mIU/L (strong recommendation) **Consider use of oral LT4** where TSH is between 2.5 and the 10 mIU/L (weak recommendation) Do not use LT4 where TSH is within the trimester-specific reference range (strong recommendation)
Assisted reproduction	–	**Recommends use of oral LT4** to reduce TSH to below 2.5 mIU/L in women with SCH undergoing in vitro fertilisation or intracytoplasmic sperm injection (strong recommendation)
Breastfeeding	–	**Treat subclinical hypothyroidism** in women wishing to breastfeed postpartum (weak recommendation)

Recommendations are abbreviated and paraphrased for clarity: see the full guidelines. *SCH* subclinical hypothyroidism, *TSH* thyrotropin, *TPO-Ab* anti-thyroid peroxidise antibody. Compiled from Refs. [14, 48]

5 Conclusions

Overt hypothyroidism must be managed effectively with oral LT4 during pregnancy, with increases in the dose made to match the changing requirements for LT4 as the pregnancy progresses. The management of subclinical hypothyroidism remains a matter for debate and further research. Clear and consistent evidence for improved pregnancy outcomes with LT4 in thyroid Ab-negative women is scarce. The presence of thyroid autoimmunity increases the risk of adverse pregnancy outcomes and is strongly associated with some causes of infertility. LT4 therapy may have a role in these patients especially those undergoing a hyperstimulation protocol as part of ART. Emerging evidence suggests that ICSI may be a particularly suitable mode of ART for women receiving LT4 for autoimmune hypothyroidism.

References

1. Korevaar TIM, Medici M, Visser TJ, Peeters RP. Thyroid disease in pregnancy: new insights in diagnosis and clinical management. Nat Rev Endocrinol. 2017;13:610–22.
2. Stagnaro-Green A, Pearce E. Thyroid disorders in pregnancy. Nat Rev Endocrinol. 2012;8:650–8.
3. Sahay RK, Sri NV. Hypothyroidism in pregnancy. Indian J Endocrinol Metab. 2012;16:364–70.
4. Loh JA, Wartofsky L, Jonklaas J, Burman KD. The magnitude of increased levothyroxine requirements in hypothyroid pregnant women depends upon the etiology of the hypothyroidism. Thyroid. 2009;19:269–75.
5. Kothari A, Girling J. Hypothyroidism in pregnancy: pre-pregnancy thyroid status influences gestational thyroxine requirements. BJOG. 2008;115:1704–8.
6. Kashi Z, Bahar A, Akha O, Hassanzade S, Esmaeilisaraji L, Hamzehgardeshi Z. Levothyroxine dosage requirement during pregnancy in well-controlled hypothyroid women: a longitudinal study. Glob J Health Sci. 2015;8:227–33.
7. Alexander EK, Marqusee E, Lawrence J, Jarolim P, Fischer GA, Larsen PR. Timing and magnitude of increases in levothyroxine requirements during pregnancy in women with hypothyroidism. N Engl J Med. 2004;351:241–9.
8. Neelaveni K, Sahay R, Hari Kumar KVS. Levothyroxine dosing after delivery in women diagnosed with hypothyroidism during pregnancy-a retrospective, observational study. Indian J Endocrinol Metab. 2019;23:238–41.
9. Busnelli A, Vannucchi G, Paffoni A, et al. Levothyroxine dose adjustment in hypothyroid women achieving pregnancy through IVF. Eur J Endocrinol. 2015;173:417–24.
10. Poppe K, Velkeniers B, Glinoer D. The role of thyroid autoimmunity in fertility and pregnancy. Nat Clin Pract Endocrinol Metab. 2008;4:394–405.
11. Korevaar TIM, Derakhshan A, Taylor PN, et al. Association of thyroid function test abnormalities and thyroid autoimmunity with preterm birth: a systematic review and meta-analysis. JAMA. 2019;322:632–41.
12. Nazarpour S, Tehrani R, Amiri M, et al. Maternal urinary iodine concentration and pregnancy outcomes: Tehran Thyroid and Pregnancy Study. Biol Trace Elem Res. 2020;194:348–59.
13. Taylor PN, Minassian C, Rehman A, et al. TSH levels and risk of miscarriage in women on long-term levothyroxine: a community-based study. J Clin Endocrinol Metab. 2014;99:3895–902.
14. Alexander EK, Pearce EN, Brent GA, et al. 2017 Guidelines of the American Thyroid Association for the diagnosis and management of thyroid disease during pregnancy and the postpartum. Thyroid. 2017;27:315–89.
15. Kim CH, Ahn JW, Kang SP, Kim SH, Chae HD, Kang BM. Effect of levothyroxine treatment on in vitro fertilization and pregnancy outcome in infertile women with subclinical hypothyroidism undergoing in vitro fertilization/intracytoplasmic sperm injection. Fertil Steril. 2011;95:1650–4.
16. Nazarpour S, Ramezani Tehrani F, Amiri M, Bidhendi Yarandi R, Azizi F. Levothyroxine treatment and pregnancy outcomes in women with subclinical hypothyroidism: a systematic review and meta-analysis. Arch Gynecol Obstet. 2019;300:805–19.
17. Maraka S, Singh Ospina NM, O'Keeffe DT, et al. Effects of increasing levothyroxine on pregnancy outcomes in women with uncontrolled hypothyroidism. Clin Endocrinol (Oxf). 2017;86:150–5.
18. Stagnaro-Green A, Roman SH, Cobin RH, el-Harazy E, Alvarez-Marfany M, Davies TF. Detection of at-risk pregnancy by means of highly sensitive assays for thyroid autoantibodies. JAMA. 1990;264:1422–5.
19. Chen L, Hu R. Thyroid autoimmunity and miscarriage: a meta-analysis. Clin Endocrinol (Oxf). 2011;74:513–9.
20. Velkeniers B, Van Meerhaeghe A, Poppe K, Unuane D, Tournaye H, Haentjens P. Levothyroxine treatment and pregnancy outcome in women with subclinical hypothyroidism undergoing assisted reproduction technologies: systematic review and meta-analysis of RCTs. Hum Reprod Update. 2013;19:251–8.

21. Thangaratinam S, Tan A, Knox E, Kilby MD, Franklyn J, Coomarasamy A. Association between thyroid autoantibodies and miscarriage and preterm birth: meta-analysis of evidence. BMJ. 2011;342:d2616.
22. Busnelli A, Paffoni A, Fedele L, Somigliana E. The impact of thyroid autoimmunity on IVF/ICSI outcome: a systematic review and meta-analysis. Hum Reprod Update. 2016;22:775–90.
23. Sitoris G, Veltri F, Kleynen P, et al. The impact of thyroid disorders on clinical pregnancy outcomes in a real-world study setting. Thyroid. 2020;30:106–15.
24. Rao M, Zeng Z, Zhao S, Tang L. Effect of levothyroxine supplementation on pregnancy outcomes in women with subclinical hypothyroidism and thyroid autoimmunity undergoing in vitro fertilization/intracytoplasmic sperm injection: an updated meta-analysis of randomized controlled trials. Reprod Biol Endocrinol. 2018;16:92.
25. Rao M, Zeng Z, Zhou F, et al. Effect of levothyroxine supplementation on pregnancy loss and preterm birth in women with subclinical hypothyroidism and thyroid autoimmunity: a systematic review and meta-analysis. Hum Reprod Update. 2019;25:344–61.
26. Li J, Shen J, Qin L. Effects of levothyroxine on pregnancy outcomes in women with thyroid dysfunction: a meta-analysis of randomized controlled trials. Altern Ther Health Med. 2017;23:49–58.
27. Nazarpour S, Ramezani Tehrani F, Simbar M, Tohidi M, Alavi Majd H, Azizi F. Effects of levothyroxine treatment on pregnancy outcomes in pregnant women with autoimmune thyroid disease. Eur J Endocrinol. 2017;176:253–65.
28. Nazarpour S, Ramezani Tehrani F, Simbar M, et al. Effects of levothyroxine on pregnant women with subclinical hypothyroidism, negative for thyroid peroxidase antibodies. J Clin Endocrinol Metab. 2018;103:926–35.
29. Dhillon-Smith RK, Middleton LJ, Sunner KK, et al. Levothyroxine in women with thyroid peroxidase antibodies before conception. N Engl J Med. 2019;380:1316–25.
30. Negro R, Mangieri T, Coppola L, et al. Levothyroxine treatment in thyroid peroxidase antibody-positive women undergoing assisted reproduction technologies: a prospective study. Hum Reprod. 2005;20:1529–33.
31. Sun X, Hou N, Wang H, Ma L, Sun J, Liu Y. A meta-analysis of pregnancy outcomes with levothyroxine treatment in euthyroid women with thyroid autoimmunity. J Clin Endocrinol Metab. 2020;105:dgz217.
32. Leduc-Robert G, Iews M, Abdelkareem AO, et al. Prevalence of thyroid autoimmunity and effect of levothyroxine treatment in a cohort of 1064 patients with recurrent pregnancy loss. Reprod Biomed Online. 2020;40:582–92.
33. Bliddal S, Feldt-Rasmussen U, Rasmussen ÅK, et al. Thyroid peroxidase antibodies and prospective live birth rate: a cohort study of women with recurrent pregnancy loss. Thyroid. 2019;29:1465–74.
34. Tosun G, Kose S, İşbilen Başok B, Altunyurt S. First-trimester placental function in levothyroxine-using pregnant women: a case-control study. Gynecol Endocrinol. 2020;36:233–7.
35. Veltri F, Kleynen P, Grabczan L, et al. Pregnancy outcomes are not altered by variation in thyroid function within the normal range in women free of thyroid disease. Eur J Endocrinol. 2018;178:189–97.
36. Unuane D, Velkeniers B, Anckaert E, et al. Thyroglobulin autoantibodies: is there any added value in the detection of thyroid autoimmunity in women consulting for fertility treatment? Thyroid. 2013;23:1022–8.
37. Wang H, Gao H, Chi H, et al. Effect of levothyroxine on miscarriage among women with normal thyroid function and thyroid autoimmunity undergoing in vitro fertilization and embryo transfer: a randomized clinical trial. JAMA. 2017;318:2190–8.
38. Poppe K, Veltri F, Autin C. Does levothyroxine improve pregnancy outcomes in euthyroid women with thyroid autoimmunity undergoing assisted reproductive technology? Thyroid Res. 2018;11:7.
39. Revelli A, Casano S, Piane LD, et al. A retrospective study on IVF outcome in euthyroid patients with anti-thyroid antibodies: effects of levothyroxine, acetyl-salicylic acid and prednisolone adjuvant treatments. Reprod Biol Endocrinol. 2009;7:137.

40. Poppe K, Autin C, Veltri F, et al. Thyroid autoimmunity and intracytoplasmic sperm injection outcome: a systematic review and meta-analysis. J Clin Endocrinol Metab. 2018 (advance publication online, https://doi.org/10.1210/jc.2017-02633).
41. Poppe K, Autin C, Veltri F, et al. Thyroid disorders and in vitro outcomes of assisted reproductive technology: an unfortunate combination? Thyroid. 2020;30:1177–85.
42. Wang P, Gao J, Zhao S, Guo Y, Wang Z, Qi F. Maternal thyroxine levels during pregnancy and outcomes of cognitive development in children. Mol Neurobiol. 2016;53:2241–8.
43. Julvez J, Alvarez-Pedrerol M, Rebagliato M, et al. Thyroxine levels during pregnancy in healthy women and early child neurodevelopment. Epidemiology. 2013;24:150–7.
44. Momotani N, Iwama S, Momotani K. Neurodevelopment in children born to hypothyroid mothers restored to normal thyroxine (T_4) concentration by late pregnancy in Japan: no apparent influence of maternal T_4 deficiency. J Clin Endocrinol Metab. 2012;97:1104–8.
45. Yamamoto JM, Benham JL, Nerenberg KA, Donovan LE. Impact of levothyroxine therapy on obstetric, neonatal and childhood outcomes in women with subclinical hypothyroidism diagnosed in pregnancy: a systematic review and meta-analysis of randomised controlled trials. BMJ Open. 2018;8:e022837.
46. Stagnaro-Green A. Second trimester levothyroxine treatment for subclinical hypothyroidism or hypothyroxinaemia of pregnancy does not improve cognitive outcomes of children. Evid Based Med. 2017;22:149.
47. Nazarpour S, Ramezani Tehrani F, Sajedi F, Bidhendi Yarandi R, Azizi F. Evaluation of the impact of levothyroxine treatment on the psychomotor developmental status of three-year-old children born to mothers with mild thyroid impairment; Tehran thyroid and pregnancy study: study protocol for a randomized clinical trial. Trials. 2019;20:86.
48. Lazarus J, Brown RS, Daumerie C, et al. 2014 European thyroid association guidelines for the management of subclinical hypothyroidism in pregnancy and in children. Eur Thyroid J. 2014;3:76–94.
49. Foeller ME, Silver RM. Combination levothyroxine + liothyronine treatment in pregnancy. Obstet Gynecol Surv. 2015;70:584–6.
50. Yassa L, Marqusee E, Fawcett R, Alexander EK. Thyroid hormone early adjustment in pregnancy (the THERAPY) trial. J Clin Endocrinol Metab. 2010;95:3234–41.
51. Vaidya B, Hubalewska-Dydejczyk A, Laurberg P, Negro R, Vermiglio F, Poppe K. Treatment and screening of hypothyroidism in pregnancy: results of a European survey. Eur J Endocrinol. 2012;166:49–54.

Levothyroxine in Children

Gabriela Brenta

Thyroid hormones are essential for the development of the central nervous system early in life. Congenital hypothyroidism once caused the devastating cognitive and physical deficits of cretinism, but this condition is now detected routinely at birth using population-wide neonatal screening in most countries. Early and continuous treatment of these children with levothyroxine (LT4), according to age-specific reference ranges, ensures near-normal neuropsychological development, with preserved IQ, although the possibility of subtle residual effects on some indices of neuropsychological functioning remain an active area of research. Children who develop overt hypothyroidism also require treatment with LT4. Most children diagnosed with subclinical hypothyroidism are unlikely to require intervention with LT4, as this condition reverses spontaneously over time. These children should be monitored for possible deterioration of thyroid function in future, especially where thyroid autoimmunity is present.

1 Introduction

This chapter considers the aetiology, clinical course, and management of hypothyroidism in children. Thyroid hormones are essential for normal physical and neural development in neonates, and many countries include a measurement of thyrotropin (thyroid-stimulating hormone; TSH) in their neonatal screening programmes.

The genetic control of thyroid hormone levels appears to function similarly in children and adults [1]. Levels of thyroid hormones differ markedly with age, however. The average level of thyrotropin is high, and highly variable, compared with usual adult measurements [2, 3]. One study showed that the average thyrotropin (thyroid-stimulating hormone, TSH) level was 6.4 mIU/L at birth, declining to 5.5, 6.6, 3.8,

G. Brenta (✉)
Dr. Cesar Milstein Hospital, Buenos Aires, Argentina

© The Author(s) 2021
G. J. Kahaly (ed.), *70 Years of Levothyroxine*,
https://doi.org/10.1007/978-3-030-63277-9_5

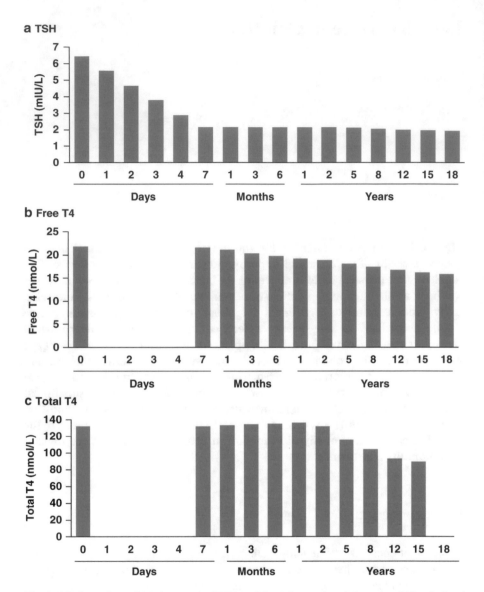

Fig. 1 Median values of (**a**) thyrotropin (TSH) and (**b, c**) free and total thyroxine (T4) calculated for children of different ages. Data were not presented between day of birth and 1 week of age for measurement of free or total T4, and for 18 years for measurement of total T4. (Drawn from data presented in Ref. [2])

2.9, and 2.1 mIU/L at 1, 2, 3, 4, and 7 days after birth, respectively [2]. Fig. 1 shows average levels of thyroid hormones from 1 month to 18 years of age [3].

Determination of reference ranges for thyroid hormones in other populations of children have confirmed the different evolution of levels of these hormones in children, compared with adults [4, 5]. These data emphasise the importance of using age-appropriate reference ranges for the diagnosis of thyroid dysfunction [5]. In general, a TSH level >5 mIU/L may be considered abnormal in children older than 1 month.

2 Overview of Hypothyroidism in Children

2.1 Congenital Hypothyroidism

The recognition of the causative role of severe, untreated hypothyroidism in the disastrous neurodevelopmental damage associated with cretinism was an important milestone in the historical development of the field of thyroidology (see chapter, "Therapeutic Use of Levothyroxine: A Historical Perspective" of this book). However, hypothyroidism may be transient in newborns identified via neonatal screening, especially when the initial TSH level is mildly elevated at diagnosis, or when relatively low LT4 doses are required for the first 2 years of life [6]. Children with congenital hypothyroidism appear to be at increased genetic risk of other adverse outcomes, including other congenital defects [7], non-alcoholic fatty liver disease [8], or urinary tract disorders [9], compared with the general population.

The optimal TSH cut-off level to diagnose congenital hypothyroidism is still a matter of debate. A study from the USA showed that TSH levels only slightly outside the reference range (e.g. ~5 mIU/L) were a poor predictor of future thyroid dysfunction, and such children need not be referred for specialist care and possible treatment [10]. However, another research group calculated that a TSH cut-off value of 6 mIU/L was optimal for identifying congenital hypothyroidism (transient or permanent) that may have required treatment [11].

2.2 Subclinical Hypothyroidism

2.2.1 Prevalence and Clinical Course

The prevalence of subclinical hypothyroidism in paediatric subjects is reported as being <2%, generally lower than the prevalence of this condition in adults [12, 13]. A large database analysis, conducted using records of more than 1 million paediatric outpatients, found that TSH was 5.5–10 mIU/L in 2.9%, and >10 mIU/L in 0.4% [14]. A recent study of more than 3 million children in Italy using administrative health databases for the years 2001–2014 found an annual prevalence of subclinical hypothyroidism (based on receipt of a low dose of LT4) of 1 case per 5000 children [15]. The annual prevalence remained relatively stable over time and tended to increase at age >10 years.

Many children with subclinical hypothyroidism revert to normal thyroid function or, at least, do not deteriorate to overt hypothyroidism [14, 16]. The analysis of >1 million children revealed that TSH reverted to within the normal range in 76% of children with initial 5.5–10 mIU/L, and in 40% of those with initial TSH >10 mIU/L [14]. The presence of thyroid autoimmunity, or higher levels of TSH at baseline, predicts a more severe clinical course, however [16–20]. In one study, the presence of Hashimoto's thyroiditis with high titres of anti-thyroglobulin antibodies was associated with a 28-fold higher risk of needing LT4 treatment vs. Hashimoto's thyroiditis patients without the presence of these antibodies [17]. Elsewhere, 63% of a population of girls with Hashimoto's thyroiditis and subclinical hypothyroidism required LT4 treatment during 5 years of follow-up, compared with 24% of girls without autoimmunity; the proportions with overt hypothyroidism at 5 years were 31% (with thyroid autoimmunity) and 12% (without thyroid autoimmunity) [21]. Children with Hashimoto's thyroiditis may still recover normal thyroid function, as shown by a study which involved withdrawal of LT4 therapy from 148 children or adolescents with this condition. One third of the population did not need re-initiation of LT4 after 2 years off-treatment [22].

2.2.2 Outcomes in Children with Subclinical Hypothyroidism

Subclinical hypothyroidism is associated with obesity in paediatric subjects [23, 24]. A retrospective study identified subclinical hypothyroidism (normal FT4, TSH 5–10 mIU/L) in 36% of a population of 215 obese children and adolescents [25]. Subjects with vs. without subclinical hypothyroidism were more insulin resistant and showed signs of atherogenic dyslipidaemia (low HDL-C, high triglycerides), but BMI was similar. Waist, BMI, LDL-C, serum triglycerides, and a measure of insulin resistance were higher, and HDL-C was lower, in 27 children (mean age 11 years) with subclinical hypothyroidism, compared with a control group [26]. Other studies have associated subclinical hypothyroidism with high blood pressure and/or other components of the metabolic syndrome in children or adolescents [23, 24, 27–29]. The TSH level correlates with insulin resistance or triglycerides in euthyroid children, also [30].

A study in 32 children with autoimmune thyroiditis and subclinical hypothyroidism (mean age 14 years) revealed increased atherogenic index, a greater thickness of epicardial fat (an emerging risk factor for metabolic dysfunction), and reduced endothelial vascular function, compared with 32 healthy matched control children [31]. A further study in 64 children also associated subclinical hypothyroidism with dyslipidaemia and increased cIMT vs. controls, although upper diagnostic limit for TSH was 20 mIU/L, and may have included children with overt hypothyroidism [32]. However, another observational study, in 110 obese children, found no correlation between TSH level and dyslipidaemia or carotid intima-media thickness, a measure of the overall burden of atherosclerosis [33].

Relatively mild neuropsychological deficits have been observed in children with subclinical hypothyroidism, relating mainly to indices of attention [12, 34, 35], or verbal memory/verbal recall [36]. Measures of intelligence of cognition were generally unaffected in these studies.

Finally, no impairment of growth or bone maturation was observed in a population of 36 children with persistent, untreated subclinical hypothyroidism followed for an average of 3.3 years [37].

2.3   Other Causes of Hypothyroidism in Children

Several other factors can produce a hypothyroid-like state in children, including consumptive hypothyroidism due to infantile hepatic hemangioma [38], older anti-epileptic drugs [39], chronic liver disease [40], or gastrointestinal disorders [41]. Other autoimmune diseases, such as type 1 diabetes or celiac disease tend to cluster with hypothyroidism in children [42–44]. Hyperprolactinaemia is also strongly associated with thyroid status: a cross-sectional study of 602 children found this disorder on 32% of children with subclinical hypothyroidism and 52% of children with overt hypothyroidism [45]. Finally, the prevalence of hypothyroidism may be higher in children with Down syndrome or Turner Syndrome, compared with the general population [46–51].

Hypothyroidism can also follow partial thyroid resection. A retrospective review of 14 aged <18 years children who had undergone hemithyroidectomy for benign thyroid nodules showed that only one patient in six needed LT4 replacement [52]. The authors suggested that these patients should be followed for sufficient time to allow natural recovery of thyroid function, before administration of LT4.

3   Effects of Levothyroxine in Children with Hypothyroidism

3.1   Congenital or Overt Hypothyroidism

Children with any form of overt hypothyroidism must be treated promptly with LT4 [53]. Treatment for congenital hypothyroidism should start within the first 2 weeks of life, and even before a confirmatory thyroid function test in more severe cases [54, 55]. A recommended starting dose is 10–15 mg/kg/day given orally, with the precise dose depending on the severity of the condition. Early and continuous treatment with LT4 effectively prevents the onset of the gross adverse effects of hypothyroidism in the brain [54]. For example, Fig. 2 shows the similar scores for measures of intelligence quotient (IQ) for children with early- and continuously treated congenital hypothyroidism, compared with euthyroid children in one study [56], and according to initial doses of LT4 in another study [57]. No behavioural abnormalities were observed between groups in the first study [56]. Optimisation of LT4 treatment is important in preserving neuropsychological outcomes in this population, as over- or under-treatment with LT4 early in life has been associated with neuropsychological or behavioural problems later on [56, 58, 59].

Severe hypothyroidism may be associated with subtle and long-lasting neuro-cognitive deficits, even when children are identified via new born screening and treated promptly with LT4. This was shown in a recent study in 30 such children aged at least 6 years, who demonstrated multiple brain white matter lesions, which correlated with deficits in language development [60]. A study from Turkey showed

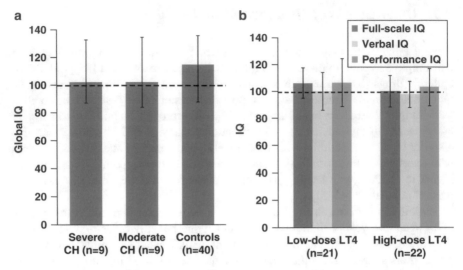

Fig. 2 Neuropsychological outcomes in children with congenital hypothyroidism (CH) treated early and continuously with levothyroxine (LT4). (**a**) *Study 1*: global intelligence quotient measured at 5.75 years of age in children with CH of varying severity, and in euthyroid control children. Children with CH received LT4 at a median dose of 12 µg/kg from a median age of 14 days. Bars show range of measurements. Differences between groups were described as being not statistically significant (the source did not provide *p* values). (Drawn from data presented in Ref. [56]). (**b**) *Study 2*: IQ measurements at 5.9 years of age in children with CH according to whether they had received a low or high dose of LT4. LT4 treatment started between 13 and 60 days after birth (mean 27 days). Low-dose LT4 = 6–<10 µg/kg/day; high-dose LT4 = 10–16 µg/kg/day. Bars are SD. There were no significant differences between low- and high-dose groups for any measure of IQ (*p* = 0.16–0.78). (Drawn from data presented in Ref. [57])

mild-to-moderate developmental delay at age 2–3 years in early-diagnosed and treated children with congenital hypothyroidism [61]. Ten-year old children with congenital hypothyroidism who were diagnosed via neonatal screening have been shown to be at risk of reduced health-related quality of life (HRQoL), and adverse perception of self-worth, compared with their euthyroid peers [62]. These deficits in QoL were independent of cognitive or neuropsychological functioning.

3.2 Subclinical Hypothyroidism

Individual studies have demonstrated that LT4 treatment reduced hypothyroid-like symptoms in children with subclinical hypothyroidism [63], or the mean anti-thyroglobulin titre in children with Hashimoto's thyroiditis [64]. Treatment of children with mild, subclinical hypothyroidism with LT4 was not disease modifying, in that it did not decrease the likelihood of an increase in TSH after treatment withdrawal [65]. There is little evidence to support improved neuropsychological outcomes with LT4 treatment in this population, however [34]. One prospective study found significantly reduced scores for verbal memory and verbal recall in 20 children with TSH 5–10 μIU/L, compared with a control group [36]. Treatment for 6 months with LT4 restored the test performance in the children with subclinical hypothyroidism to the level of controls.

Obesity is associated with hypothyroidism (especially the subclinical form) in children, as described above. A 6-month, randomised trial in 51 obese children with TSH 4–10 mIU/L (with or without abnormalities of other thyroid hormones) showed that administration of LT4 vs. no additional treatment, alongside weight loss interventions, had no significant effect on BMI or lipid abnormalities [66]. A similar study, where LT4 was or was not added to a behavioural intervention for obesity, reported similar results [67]. These data suggest there is no place for LT4 in the general management of obesity in children with TSH levels consistent with subclinical hypothyroidism. Correlations of higher TSH levels with higher BMI in hypothyroid children controlled on LT4 have been observed [68], but this association is probably not independently causative for obesity [1, 69].

Administration of LT4 to 30 children with subclinical hypothyroidism (mean age 7 years, mean TSH 8.7 mIU/L) for 6 months increased measures of left ventricular systolic performance (myocardial performance index, fraction shortening, and ejection fraction), but did not affect diastolic function (E/E' ratio) [70]. This study was uncontrolled, and these parameters were not overtly decreased before treatment, so that the clinical relevance of these findings is difficult to assess. Migraine may be a symptom of subclinical hypothyroidism, which responds to treatment with LT4 [71].

Box 1 summarises guideline recommendations for the management of subclinical hypothyroidism in children [43, 53, 69]. The majority of this population will not need active treatment, as long as thyroid hormones are within range and thyroid function is not deteriorating. The European guidance differs from the guidelines from Latin America and from the USA since it was specifically addressed for hypothyroidism in children, and it identifies the first 3 years of life as the crucial period for optimising thyroid function with LT4 (this is the time when thyroid hormones have their greatest influence on development of the brain). Monotherapy with LT4 is used exclusively: there is no role for the therapeutic use of T3 currently, as in other populations. A recent expert opinion recommends reserving LT4-based management of subclinical hypothyroidism to children with autoimmune (Hashimoto) disease, children whose thyroid function is deteriorating over time, or for children with goitre, other congenital abnormalities associated with thyroid dysfunction (Turner Syndrome or Down Syndrome) [72].

Box 1: Summary of Guidance Relating to the Use of Levothyroxine (LT4) in Children with Subclinical Hypothyroidism [46, 53, 69]

- Discuss decisions to treat or not to treat with LT4 carefully with parents/ guardians
- Most children with TSH <10 mIU/L and FT4 or TT4 within normal range will not need treatment with LT4
- Initiating LT4 is a reasonable strategy for patients with TSH >10 mIU/L, including children

    – *Especially beyond 1 month of age and who have signs and symptoms of hypothyroidism and/or risk factors for progression of thyroid dysfunction*

- Use LT4 only, there is no current role for treatment with LT3
- Consider a trial of withdrawal of LT4 at age 3 years, as development of the CNS is no longer dependent on thyroid function
- Monitor the TSH level and for thyroid autoimmunity periodically beyond age 3 years (more frequent monitoring is recommended if thyroid autoimmunity is present already)

Guidance has been adapted and combined from Latin American [46], the USA [53], and European [69] guidelines and has been paraphrased for brevity. See the full guidelines for more details

3.3   Biochemically Euthyroid Children

A randomised trial in 59 biochemically euthyroid children with Hashimoto's thyroiditis showed that treatment with LT4 (mean dose 1.6 µg/kg/day, based individually on body weight) vs. no treatment reduced thyroid volume transiently, and did not affect either thyroid function or the level of thyroid autoantibodies [73]. Observational data from 330 children with autoimmune thyroiditis and type 1 diabetes showed a reduction in antibodies in the treated cohort, suggesting a possible role for LT4 therapy in this population [74].

4   Conclusions

Thyroid hormones are essential for the development of the central nervous system early in life. Early and continuous treatment with LT4 of children with overt hypothyroidism preserves near-normal neuropsychological development. Subclinical hypothyroidism often resolves spontaneously and most children will not need LT4 treatment. However, close observation is key since some children with this condition may require LT4 to manage symptoms, or they may develop overt hypothyroidism in the future.

References

1. Nielsen TR, Appel EV, Svendstrup M, et al. A genome-wide association study of thyroid stimulating hormone and free thyroxine in Danish children and adolescents. PLoS One. 2017;12:e0174204.
2. Lem AJ, de Rijke YB, van Toor H, de Ridder MA, Visser TJ, Hokken-Koelega AC. Serum thyroid hormone levels in healthy children from birth to adulthood and in short children born small for gestational age. J Clin Endocrinol Metab. 2012;97:3170–8.
3. Kapelari K, Kirchlechner C, Högler W, Schweitzer K, Virgolini I, Moncayo R. Pediatric reference intervals for thyroid hormone levels from birth to adulthood: a retrospective study. BMC Endocr Disord. 2008;8:15.
4. Soldin OP, Jang M, Guo T, Soldin SJ. Pediatric reference intervals for free thyroxine and free triiodothyronine. Thyroid. 2009;19:699–702.
5. La'ulu SL, Rasmussen KJ, Straseski JA. Pediatric reference intervals for free thyroxine and free triiodothyronine by equilibrium dialysis-liquid chromatography-tandem mass spectrometry. J Clin Res Pediatr Endocrinol. 2016;8:26–31.
6. Kang MJ, Chung HR, Oh YJ, Shim YS, Yang S, Hwang IT. Three-year follow-up of children with abnormal newborn screening results for congenital hypothyroidism. Pediatr Neonatol. 2017;58:442–8.
7. Wędrychowicz A, Furtak A, Prośniak A, et al. Extrathyroidal congenital defects in children with congenital hypothyroidism—observations from a single paediatric centre in Central Europe with a review of literature. Pediatr Endocrinol Diabetes Metab. 2019;25:114–21.
8. Pan YW, Tsai MC, Yang YJ, Chen MY, Chen SY, Chou YY. The relationship between nonalcoholic fatty liver disease and pediatric congenital hypothyroidism patients. Kaohsiung J Med Sci. 2019;35:778–86.
9. Kumar J, Gordillo R, Kaskel FJ, Druschel CM, Woroniecki RP. Increased prevalence of renal and urinary tract anomalies in children with congenital hypothyroidism. J Pediatr. 2009;154:263–6.
10. Gammons S, Presley BK, White PC. Referrals for elevated thyroid stimulating hormone to pediatric endocrinologists. J Endocr Soc. 2019;3:2032–40.
11. Langham S, Hindmarsh P, Krywawych S, Peters C. Screening for congenital hypothyroidism: comparison of borderline screening cut-off points and the effect on the number of children treated with levothyroxine. Eur Thyroid J. 2013;2:180–6.
12. Wu T, Flowers JW, Tudiver F, Wilson JL, Punyasavatsut N. Subclinical thyroid disorders and cognitive performance among adolescents in the United States. BMC Pediatr. 2006;6:12.
13. Gallizzi R, Crisafulli C, Aversa T, et al. Subclinical hypothyroidism in children: is it always subclinical? Ital J Pediatr. 2018;44:25.
14. Lazar L, Frumkin RB, Battat E, Lebenthal Y, Phillip M, Meyerovitch J. Natural history of thyroid function tests over 5 years in a large pediatric cohort. J Clin Endocrinol Metab. 2009;94:1678–82.
15. Greggio NA, Rossi E, Calabria S, et al. Subclinical hypothyroidism in paediatric population treated with levothyroxine: a real-world study on 2001-2014 Italian administrative data. Endocr Connect. 2017;6:367–74.

16. Valenzise M, Aversa T, Zirilli G, et al. Analysis of the factors affecting the evolution over time of subclinical hypothyroidism in children. Ital J Pediatr. 2017;43:2.
17. Lee YJ, Jung SY, Jung HW, et al. Unfavorable course of subclinical hypothyroidism in children with Hashimoto's thyroiditis compared to those with isolated non-autoimmune hyperthyrotropinemia. J Korean Med Sci. 2017;32:124–9.
18. Radetti G, Maselli M, Buzi F, et al. The natural history of the normal/mild elevated TSH serum levels in children and adolescents with Hashimoto's thyroiditis and isolated hyperthyrotropinaemia: a 3-year follow-up. Clin Endocrinol (Oxf). 2012;76:394–8.
19. Aversa T, Valenzise M, Corrias A, et al. Underlying Hashimoto's thyroiditis negatively affects the evolution of subclinical hypothyroidism in children irrespective of other concomitant risk factors. Thyroid. 2015;25:183–7.
20. Aversa T, Corrias A, Salerno M, et al. Five-year prospective evaluation of thyroid function test evolution in children with hashimoto's thyroiditis presenting with either euthyroidism or subclinical hypothyroidism. Thyroid. 2016;26:1450–6.
21. Wasniewska M, Aversa T, Salerno M, et al. Five-year prospective evaluation of thyroid function in girls with subclinical mild hypothyroidism of different etiology. Eur J Endocrinol. 2015;173:801–8.
22. Radetti G, Salerno M, Guzzetti C, et al. Thyroid function in children and adolescents with Hashimoto's thyroiditis after l-thyroxine discontinuation. Endocr Connect. 2017;6:206–12.
23. Cerbone M, Capalbo D, Wasniewska M, et al. Cardiovascular risk factors in children with long-standing untreated idiopathic subclinical hypothyroidism. J Clin Endocrinol Metab. 2014;99:2697–703.
24. Zhang J, Jiang R, Li L, Li P, Li X, Wang Z, et al. Serum thyrotropin is positively correlated with the metabolic syndrome components of obesity and dyslipidemia in Chinese adolescents. Int J Endocrinol. 2014;2014:289503.
25. Kara O. Influence of subclinical hypothyroidism on metabolic parameters in obese children and adolescents. Clin Exp Pediatr. 2020;63:110–4.
26. Yadav Y, Saikia UK, Sarma D, Hazarika M. Cardiovascular risk factors in children and adolescents with subclinical hypothyroidism. Indian J Endocrinol Metab. 2017;21:823–9.
27. Chen H, Xi Q, Zhang H, et al. Investigation of thyroid function and blood pressure in school-aged subjects without overt thyroid disease. Endocrine. 2012;41:122–9.
28. Ittermann T, Thamm M, Wallaschofski H, Rettig R, Völzke H. Serum thyroid stimulating hormone levels are associated with blood pressure in children and adolescents. Clin Endocrinol Metab. 2012;97:828–84.
29. Cerbone M, Capalbo D, Wasniewska M, et al. Effects of L-thyroxine treatment on early markers of atherosclerotic disease in children with subclinical hypothyroidism. Eur J Endocrinol. 2016;175:11–9.
30. Nader NS, Bahn RS, Johnson MD, Weaver AL, Singh R, Kumar S. Relationships between thyroid function and lipid status or insulin resistance in a pediatric population. Thyroid. 2010;20:1333–9.
31. Farghaly HS, Metwalley KA, Raafat DM, Algowhary M, Said GM. Epicardial fat thickness in children with subclinical hypothyroidism and its relationship to subclinical atherosclerosis: a pilot study. Horm Res Paediatr. 2019;92:99–105.
32. Unal E, Akın A, Yıldırım R, Demir V, Yildiz İ, Haspolat YK. Association of subclinical hypothyroidism with dyslipidemia and increased carotid intima-media thickness in children. J Clin Res Pediatr Endocrinol. 2017;9:144–9.
33. Rumińska M, Witkowska-Sędek E, Majcher A, Brzewski M, Krawczyk M, Pyrżak B. Serum TSH level in obese children and its correlations with atherogenic lipid indicators and carotid intima media thickness. J Ultrason. 2018;18:296–301.
34. Aijaz NJ, Flaherty EM, Preston T, Bracken SS, Lane AH, Wilson TA. Neurocognitive function in children with compensated hypothyroidism: lack of short term effects on or off thyroxin. BMC Endocr Disord. 2006;6:2.

35. Ergür AT, Taner Y, Ata E, Melek E, Bakar EE, Sancak T. Neurocognitive functions in children and adolescents with subclinical hypothyroidism. J Clin Res Pediatr Endocrinol. 2012;4:21–4.
36. Sangün Ö, Demirci S, Dündar N, et al. The effects of six-month L-Thyroxine treatment on cognitive functions and event-related brain potentials in children with subclinical hypothyroidism. J Clin Res Pediatr Endocrinol. 2015;7:102–8.
37. Cerbone M, Bravaccio C, Capalbo D, et al. Linear growth and intellectual outcome in children with long-term idiopathic subclinical hypothyroidism. Eur J Endocrinol. 2011;164:591–7.
38. Weber Pasa M, Selbach Scheffel R, Borsatto Zanella A, Maia AL, Dora JM. Consumptive hypothyroidism: case report of hepatic hemangioendotheliomas successfully treated with vincristine and systematic review of the syndrome. Eur Thyroid J. 2017;6:321–7.
39. Elshorbagy HH, Barseem NF, Suliman HA, et al. The impact of antiepileptic drugs on thyroid function in children with epilepsy: new versus old. Iran J Child Neurol. 2020;14:31–41.
40. Ön ŞŞ, Acar S, Demir K, et al. Evaluation of thyroid function tests in children with chronic liver diseases. J Clin Res Pediatr Endocrinol. 2020;12:143–9.
41. Passos ACV, Barros F, Damiani D, et al. Hypothyroidism associated with short bowel syndrome in children: a report of six cases. Arch Endocrinol Metab. 2018;62:655–60.
42. Ridha MF, Al Zubaidi MA. Thyroid auto immune antibodies in children with type-I diabetes mellitus in relation to diabetes control. Pak J Med Sci. 2019;35:969–73.
43. Sharma B, Nehara HR, Saran S, Bhavi VK, Singh AK, Mathur SK. Coexistence of autoimmune disorders and type 1 diabetes mellitus in children: an observation from western part of India. Indian J Endocrinol Metab. 2019;23:22–6.
44. Kakleas K, Paschali E, Kefalas N, et al. Factors for thyroid autoimmunity in children and adolescents with type 1 diabetes mellitus. Ups J Med Sci. 2009;114:214–20.
45. Sharma N, Dutta D, Sharma LK. Hyperprolactinemia in children with subclinical hypothyroidism. J Clin Res Pediatr Endocrinol. 2017;9:350–4.
46. Brenta G, Vaisman M, Sgarbi JA, et al. Clinical practice guidelines for the management of hypothyroidism. Arq Bras Endocrinol Metabol. 2013;57:265–91.
47. Pierce MJ, LaFranchi SH, Pinter JD. Characterization of thyroid abnormalities in a large cohort of children with Down syndrome. Horm Res Paediatr. 2017;87:170–8.
48. Kowalczyk K, Pukajło K, Malczewska A, Król-Chwastek A, Barg E. L-thyroxine therapy and growth processes in children with Down syndrome. Adv Clin Exp Med. 2013;22:85–92.
49. De Sanctis V, Khater D. Autoimmune diseases in Turner syndrome: an overview. Acta Biomed. 2019;90:341–4.
50. Liu MY, Lee CT, Lee NC, et al. Thyroid disorders in Taiwanese children with Down syndrome: the experience of a single medical center. J Formos Med Assoc. 2020;119:345–9.
51. Yaqoob M, Manzoor J, Hyder SN, Sadiq M. Congenital heart disease and thyroid dysfunction in Down syndrome reported at Children's Hospital, Lahore, Pakistan. Turk J Pediatr. 2019;61:915–24.
52. Chen J, Hou S, Li X, Yang J. Management of subclinical and overt hypothyroidism following hemithyroidectomy in children and adolescents: a pilot study. Front Pediatr. 2019;7:396.
53. Jonklaas J, Bianco AC, Bauer AJ, et al. Guidelines for the treatment of hypothyroidism: prepared by the American Thyroid Association task force on thyroid hormone replacement. Thyroid. 2014;24:1670–751.
54. Léger J, Olivieri A, Donaldson M, et al. European Society for Paediatric Endocrinology consensus guidelines on screening, diagnosis, and management of congenital hypothyroidism. J Clin Endocrinol Metab. 2014;99:363–84.
55. Rastogi MV, LaFranchi SH. Congenital hypothyroidism. Orphanet J Rare Dis. 2010;5:17.
56. Simoneau-Roy J, Marti S, Deal C, Huot C, Robaey P, Van Vliet G. Cognition and behavior at school entry in children with congenital hypothyroidism treated early with high-dose levothyroxine. J Pediatr. 2004;144:747–52.
57. Seo MK, Yoon JS, So CH, Lee HS, Hwang JS. Intellectual development in preschool children with early treated congenital hypothyroidism. Ann Pediatr Endocrinol Metab. 2017;22:102–7.

58. García Morales L, Rodríguez Arnao MD, Rodríguez Sánchez A, Dulín Íñiguez E, Álvarez González MA. Sustained attention in school-age children with congenital hypothyroidism: influence of episodes of overtreatment in the first three years of life. Neurologia. 2017. pii: S0213-4853(17)30299-2.
59. Bongers-Schokking JJ, Resing WCM, Oostdijk W, de Rijke YB, de Muinck Keizer-Schrama SMPF. Relation between early over- and undertreatment and behavioural problems in preadolescent children with congenital hypothyroidism. Horm Res Paediatr. 2018;90:247–56.
60. Cooper HE, Kaden E, Halliday LF, et al. White matter microstructural abnormalities in children with severe congenital hypothyroidism. Neuroimage Clin. 2019;24:101980.
61. Baysal BT, Baysal B, Genel F, et al. Neurodevelopmental outcome of children with congenital hypothyroidism diagnosed in a national screening program in Turkey. Indian Pediatr. 2017;54:381–4.
62. van der Sluijs VL, Kempers MJ, Maurice-Stam H, Last BF, Vulsma T, Grootenhuis MA. Health-related quality of life and self-worth in 10-year old children with congenital hypothyroidism diagnosed by neonatal screening. Child Adolesc Psychiatry Ment Health. 2012;6:32.
63. Çatlı G, Anık A, Ünver Tuhan H, Böber E, Abacı A. The effect of L-thyroxine treatment on hypothyroid symptom scores and lipid profile in children with subclinical hypothyroidism. J Clin Res Pediatr Endocrinol. 2014;6:238–44.
64. Özen S, Berk Ö, Şimşek DG, Darcan S. Clinical course of Hashimoto's thyroiditis and effects of levothyroxine therapy on the clinical course of the disease in children and adolescents. J Clin Res Pediatr Endocrinol. 2011;3:192–7.
65. Wasniewska M, Corrias A, Aversa T, et al. Comparative evaluation of therapy with L-thyroxine versus no treatment in children with idiopathic and mild subclinical hypothyroidism. Horm Res Paediatr. 2012;77:376–81.
66. Kumar S, Dayal D, Attri S, Gupta A, Bhalla A. Levothyroxine supplementation for obesity-associated thyroid dysfunction in children: a prospective, randomized, case control study. Pediatr Endocrinol Diabetes Metab. 2019;25:107–13.
67. Matusik P, Gawlik A, Januszek-Trzciakowska A, Malecka-Tendera E. Isolated subclinical hyperthyrotropinemia in obese children: does levothyroxine (LT4) improve weight reduction during combined behavioral therapy? Int J Endocrinol. 2015;2015:792509.
68. Shaoba A, Basu S, Mantis S, Minutti C. Serum thyroid-stimulating hormone levels and body mass index percentiles in children with primary hypothyroidism on levothyroxine replacement. J Clin Res Pediatr Endocrinol. 2017;9:337–43.
69. Lazarus J, Brown RS, Daumerie C, Hubalewska-Dydejczyk A, Negro R, Vaidya B. 2014 European Thyroid Association guidelines for the management of subclinical hypothyroidism in pregnancy and in children. Eur Thyroid J. 2014;3:76–94.
70. Banu Rupani N, Alijanpour M, Babazadeh K, Hajian-Tilaki K, Moadabdoost F. Effect of levothyroxine on cardiac function in children with subclinical hypothyroidism: a quasi-experimental study. Caspian J Intern Med. 2019;10:332–8.
71. Mirouliaei M, Fallah R, Bashardoost N, Partovee M, Ordooei M. Efficacy of levothyroxine in migraine headaches in children with subclinical hypothyroidism. Iran J Child Neurol. 2012;6:23–6.
72. Crisafulli G, Aversa T, Zirilli G, et al. Subclinical hypothyroidism in children: when a replacement hormonal treatment might be advisable. Front Endocrinol (Lausanne). 2019;10:109.
73. Dörr HG, Bettendorf M, Binder G, et al. Levothyroxine treatment of euthyroid children with autoimmune Hashimoto thyroiditis: results of a multicenter, randomized, controlled trial. Horm Res Paediatr. 2015;84:266–74.
74. Korzeniowska K, Jarosz-Chobot P, Szypowska A, et al. L-thyroxine stabilizes autoimmune inflammatory process in euthyroid nongoitrous children with Hashimoto's thyroiditis and type 1 diabetes mellitus. J Clin Res Pediatr Endocrinol. 2013;5:240–4.

Levothyroxine in the Older Patient

Salman Razvi

Levels of the pituitary hormone thyrotropin (thyroid-stimulating hormone, TSH) tend to run higher in older individuals than in younger adults. As TSH is used to guide replacement with levothyroxine (LT4), older patients may be at risk of over treatment if TSH levels towards the lower part of the standard adult reference range are aimed for. Recent randomised clinical trials have not demonstrated clinical benefit from the use of LT4 in older patients with subclinical hypothyroidism (diagnosed and treated according to standard, adult TSH reference ranges). The results of the recent Study of Optimal Replacement of Thyroxine in the Elderly (SORTED 1) feasibility trial suggest that older hypothyroid patients can be treated using a higher than usual target range for TSH with no apparent adverse effects, at least over the short term.

1 Thyroid Homeostasis in Older Individuals

1.1 Thyroid Homeostasis

Hypothyroidism is diagnosed when serum thyrotropin (thyroid-stimulating hormone or TSH) is elevated and thyroid hormones are low. The incidence of hypothyroidism increases with age. The reference range limits for serum TSH and thyroid hormones are calculated from measurements obtained from all age groups. However, both the median and 97.5th centile values for TSH increase with age (Fig. 1) [1]. Several studies from various parts of the world have confirmed the increase in serum TSH concentrations with ageing [2–6].

S. Razvi (✉)
Translational and Clinical Research Institute, University of Newcastle, Newcastle-upon-Tyne, UK
e-mail: salman.razvi@newcastle.ac.uk

© The Author(s) 2021
G. J. Kahaly (ed.), *70 Years of Levothyroxine*,
https://doi.org/10.1007/978-3-030-63277-9_6

75

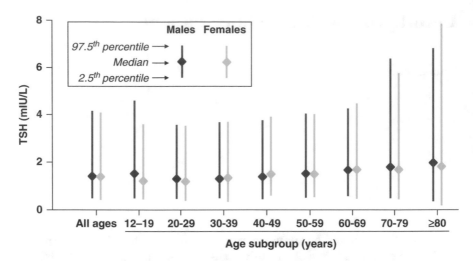

Fig. 1 Medians and 2.5th–97.5th percentile reference ranges for thyrotropin (TSH) according to age in healthy subjects from a large (*n* = 13,344) population-based study in the USA. Subjects with risk factors for thyroid dysfunction such as pregnancy, oestrogens, androgens, lithium, antithyroid antibodies, and treated thyroid disease were excluded. (Drawn from data presented in Ref. [1])

A study of ambulatory older individuals found that 1 in 40 people had low levels of circulating free thyroxine (FT4) index although thyrotropin levels were normal [7]. A comparison of six of these subjects (mean age 69 years) with six age- and gender-matched subjects with normal FT4 index (also with a normal thyrotropin level) showed that pituitary or hypothalamic dysfunction, pituitary thyrotropin reserve, thyroid reserve, and the biological actions of secreted thyrotropin, did not differ between these groups [7]. Accordingly, the authors concluded that this functional hypothyroidism in some older patients was due to a resetting of the hypothalamic-pituitary-thyroid feedback axis. The mechanisms underlying the increase in TSH with age remain to be elucidated. It does appear, however, that TSH secretion in older people is increased without any change in its bioactivity [8].

1.2   Thyroid Hormone Levels and Clinical Outcomes

Lower TSH or higher FT4 levels, including variations of these hormones within the normal range, have been associated with increased risk of mortality [9–12], major adverse cardiovascular events (including myocardial infarction) [13], heart failure [14], frailty [15], and dementia [16, 17] in older populations. Conversely, low-normal FT4 was associated with better mobility and less fatigue, compared with higher levels of FT4, in a study of 602 older euthyroid individuals [18].

Not all studies have associated higher FT4 levels within the normal range with adverse outcomes in older patients, however. Higher thyrotropin and lower FT4 in hospitalised older patients was associated with an increased risk of a composite of morbidity/mortality outcomes (death, admission to the intensive care unit, or hospital stay >18 days) in a retrospective study [19]. Another study found a higher rate of cognitive decline over time in older women with low-normal vs. high-normal, FT4 [20]. A population-based study demonstrated no association between FT4 levels and cognitive decline in a cohort born in 1912–1914 [10].

Some of these studies suggested little or no significant effect of modest increases in TSH (consistent with subclinical hypothyroidism) on outcomes in this population, even where higher FT4 was associated with an adverse prognosis [12, 14, 17]. Higher TSH in 85 year-old individuals was associated with reduced mortality in the Leiden 85+ study though the authors emphasised the need for further data to corroborate this finding [10]. Another study of a larger number of 85-year-old individuals followed up for a longer period of time than the Leiden study did not confirm the protective association of high TSH with mortality in this age group but nevertheless confirmed that a slightly raised serum TSH was not associated with adverse outcomes [4]. Elsewhere, the risk of heart failure was only increased if TSH was unequivocally abnormal (<0.1 or >10 mIU/L) [14]. A meta-analysis concluded that the excess risk of adverse cardiovascular outcomes in older patients with subclinical hypothyroidism was small, with minimal increased risk in studies of higher quality (relative risks 1.2–1.8 vs. euthyroid individuals) [21]. A second meta-analysis found no association between subclinical hypothyroidism and adverse cardiovascular outcomes in older patients [22].

2 Therapeutic Use of Levothyroxine in Older Patients with Hypothyroidism

2.1 Analyses from Randomised, Placebo-Controlled Trials

The Thyroid Hormone Replacement for Untreated Older Adults with Subclinical Hypothyroidism Trial (TRUST) randomised 737 adults aged ≥65 years with thyrotropin 4.6–<20 mIU/L and normal FT4 to double-blind treatment with levothyroxine (LT4) or placebo for 1 year [23, 24]. As expected, mean thyrotropin was lower in the LT4 group (3.6 mIU/L) compared with the placebo group (5.5 mIU/L) at study end. However, there was no effect on the co-primary endpoints in this study (change from baseline in two validated questionnaires specific to thyroid dysfunction: Hypothyroid Symptoms and Tiredness, and the Thyroid-Related Quality-of-Life Patient-Reported Outcome Questionnaire), or on other secondary outcomes. The TRUST trial has been criticised for recruiting participants with mostly low symptom burden [25]. Therefore, it is interesting that a *post hoc* analysis in subjects with more pronounced symptoms of hypothyroidism at baseline produced a similar lack of clinical benefit of LT4 treatment [26]. Additional sub-analysis from TRUST found no effect of LT4 treatment on cardiac function [27] or bone metabolism [28] in this population.

Pooling the data from two randomised trials, including a subgroup from TRUST, involving a total of 251 patients with subclinical hypothyroidism aged ≥80 years also found no significant effect of LT4 on thyroid symptoms or fatigue, relative to placebo [29]. Administration of LT4 for 1 year to patients aged ≥65 years in the primary care setting had no significant effect on cognitive function [30]. A randomised trial in outpatients aged 55 years or over reported a nominally significant effect of LT4 treatment on a composite memory score though there were no benefits of treatments relating to other endpoints, or to health-related quality of life [31]. A meta-analysis published in 2018, which included two studies in patients aged >65 years with subclinical hypothyroidism also found no evidence of clinical benefit arising from intervention with LT4 [32].

Hypothyroidism has been associated with an adverse cardiovascular prognosis in some studies (see chapter, "Levothyroxine and the Heart"). Randomisation of 185 patients with subclinical hypothyroidism in a nested subgroup of participants within the TRUST trial aged ≥65 years to LT4 vs. placebo for an average of 18 months had no significant effect on carotid intima-media thickness (a measure of the overall burden of atherosclerosis), however [33].

2.2 Observational Studies of Levothyroxine in Older Patients with Hypothyroidism

Observational data in subjects with subclinical hypothyroidism (diagnosed using a cut-off for thyrotropin of 8 mIU/L) showed that a similar overall improvement from baseline in health-related quality of life occurred following LT4 treatment in younger (<40 years) and older (>60 years) patients [34]. Both age groups benefitted from improvements in "Emotional Susceptibility" and "Impaired Daily Life" domains; older patients additionally improved their score for "Tiredness" and younger patients improved their score for "Cognitive Complaints". A recent study that included 24 patients with hypothyroidism who were aged ≥65 years and already receiving stable doses of LT4 involved increasing the dose of LT4 by 12.5 mg/day (irrespective of the previous dose) in a single-blind manner for 3 months [35]. This change was sufficient to reduce mean thyrotropin from 1.95 to 0.47 mIU/L. The period of administration of the higher LT4 dose was accompanied by a significant improvement in the Geriatric Depression Scale score, including in patients with a score consistent with clinical depression at baseline, without inducing symptoms of hyperthyroidism. However, the impact of higher doses of LT4 in this age group on long-term outcomes, particularly the risk of atrial fibrillation and osteoporosis, is unknown.

Any severity of hyperthyroidism increases the risk of bone fractures [36], which is a particular concern for the elderly who may be already at risk of age-related osteoporosis [37]. Treatment of women aged ≥65 years with LT4 at a daily dose >150 μg/day was associated with increased fracture risk in an observational study, with the highest risk in women already receiving treatment for osteoporosis [38]. A case-control study in subjects aged ≥70 years also found a dose-related increase in the risk of fractures associated with LT4 treatment [39]. One potential mechanism for the observed adverse events may be due to the risk of inadvertent over-treatment with LT4. In a community-based cohort study, iatrogenic thyrotoxicosis accounted for approximately half of low TSH events, with the highest rates among older women, who are vulnerable to atrial fibrillation and osteoporosis [40]. No evidence of any differences in long-term health outcomes are observed when thyrotropin concentrations are maintained within the reference range [41]. Chapter "Levothyroxine and Bone" provides a fuller account of the effects of LT4 on bone health.

2.3 Managing Elderly Patients with Hypothyroidism: Implications of the SORTED 1 Trial

The studies reviewed above suggest that the clinical sequelae of hypothyroidism, particularly the subclinical form, appear to be less severe in older vs. younger patients. The randomised evaluations of LT4 have not provided unequivocal evidence for benefit of intervention with LT4 in older patients, especially those with subclinical hypothyroidism [23, 24, 26–29]. It is important to remember that the diagnosis of hypothyroidism and the titration of the LT4 dose were guided in these studies by standard reference ranges for thyrotropin in adults. Given the shift towards higher levels of thyrotropin in elderly populations, the population of TRUST and similar studies probably included individuals who had high TSH relative to the standard adult reference range, who would have been classified as euthyroid using a more age-appropriate reference range [32].

The Study of Optimal Replacement of Thyroxine in the Elderly (SORTED1) study evaluated the clinical consequences of using LT4 to control the level of thyrotropin within a higher range than the usual reference range used to guide LT4 therapy in adults [42–44]. This trial was conducted in 48 elderly (≥80 years) patients with pre-existing hypothyroidism whose thyrotropin was well controlled as per the usual local adult reference range (0.4–4.0 mIU/L). The patients were randomised in a single-blind manner to continuing treatment guided by the standard reference range, or by a higher range (4.1–8.0 mIU/L) for 6 months.

As expected, the mean thyrotropin level (±SD) was higher at 6 months in the higher range group (6.6 ± 2.9 mIU/L) than in the standard range group (1.4 ± 1.0 mIU/L); corresponding mean values of other hormones were 16.0 ± 2.5 and 19.4 ± 3.5 pmol/L, respectively, for FT4 and 3.5 ± 0.5 and 3.9 ± 0.4 pmol/L, respectively, for FT3. The mean FT3/FT4 ratio was similar in the higher range (0.23 ± 0.04) and standard range (0.21 ± 0.05) groups.

There were no clinically significant differences between groups for mean values of lipid parameters, blood pressures, weight, pulse rate, and a bone resorption marker at study end (Fig. 2). In addition, small and similar changes in group occurred in scores on questionnaires that measured generic and thyroid dysfunction-specific quality of life (EQ-5D and ThyDQoL), or on the risk of falling (falls risk assessment test) or mobility (timed up and go test). The most common all-cause adverse events (AE) in the standard and higher range groups were "Feeling more tired" (38% and 50%, respectively) and "Problems with balance or mobility" (17% in each group). No other AE occurred in more than two patients in either group.

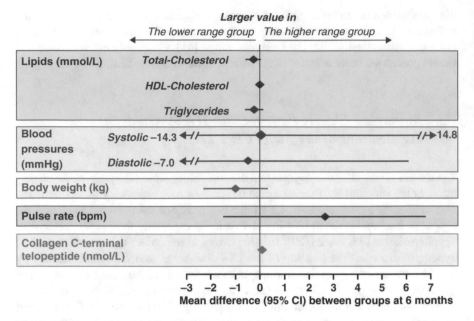

Fig. 2 Effects of randomisation of elderly subjects with subclinical hypothyroidism to a higher or lower target range for thyrotropin on cardiovascular risk factors and a marker of bone resorption in the SORTED 1 Trial. Formal statistical testing was not carried out in this trial, but differences may be considered to be not statistically significant as 95%CI for mean differences between groups overlap zero for every parameter. *HDL* high density lipoprotein. See text for definitions of higher and lower range groups. (Drawn from data presented in Ref. [44])

3   Conclusions

Thyrotropin levels shift towards higher concentrations in older individuals but current reference ranges are applied uniformly across all age groups. Hence, a significant number of people, particularly in the older age group, are diagnosed with subclinical hypothyroidism and a proportion of these are treated with LT4. The long-term health outcomes and cost-effectiveness of treatment in this particular group of patients is unknown. Furthermore, it also remains unclear whether a higher thyrotropin reference range should be aimed for in older patients on LT4 therapy.

The SORTED 1 trial demonstrated that titrating LT4 therapy to a higher than usual reference range in elderly patients may not adversely affect symptoms of hypothyroidism, or impair quality of life. Moreover, this trial has shown that a suitably powered long-term study is feasible, in order to verify these findings.

Current guidelines for the management of hypothyroidism in adults date back to 2014, or earlier [45, 46]. These guidelines acknowledge the shift towards higher levels of thyrotropin as people age (Box 1), as well as the possibility of accepting a higher target value for thyrotropin. There is no unequivocal recommendation to use age-specific reference ranges for thyrotropin in elderly patients with hypothyroidism, however. There is growing recognition, though, that the TSH reference range does need to appropriately reflect the age of the individual [47]. The results of recent randomised trials, including SORTED 1 and TRUST, will inform future guidance on the management of the elderly patient with hypothyroidism, probably leading to a less intensive application of LT4 and acceptance of a higher range of thyrotropin levels in elderly patients.

Box 1: Key Recommendations from the USA [45] and European [46] Guidelines on the General Approach for the Management of Hypothyroidism in Elderly Patients

- Thyrotropin levels tend to be higher in elderly vs. younger people with hypothyroidism, and a higher than usual target level of thyrotropin may be acceptable for an elderly patient [45, 46].
- The dose of LT4 to control the thyrotropin level is lower, on average, in older vs. younger subjects, due in part to a lower muscle mass in this population [45].
- Extra vigilance for interference of other medications with the effects of LT4 is necessary for the elderly population, who may be receiving multiple other treatments for comorbid conditions [45].
- Avoidance of iatrogenic thyrotoxicosis due to over treatment with LT4 is a clinical priority in elderly patients with hypothyroidism, especially given the association of higher FT4 levels with adverse outcomes, described above [45].
- Consider monitoring, rather than intervening with LT4, for very elderly (>80 years) patients with subclinical hypothyroidism [46].
- Consider a "start low, go slow" approach to administering LT4 to elderly patients [45, 46].

References

1. Hollowell JG, Staehling NW, Flanders WD, et al. Serum TSH, T(4), and thyroid antibodies in the United States population (1988 to 1994): National Health and Nutrition Examination Survey (NHANES III). J Clin Endocrinol Metab. 2002;87:489–99.
2. Ceresini G, Lauretani F, Maggio M, et al. Thyroid function abnormalities and cognitive impairment in elderly people: results of the Invecchiare in Chianti study. J Am Geriatr Soc. 2009;57:89–93.
3. Yeap BB. Hormones and health outcomes in aging men. Exp Gerontol. 2013;48:677–81.
4. Pearce SH, Razvi S, Yadegarfar ME, et al. Serum thyroid function, mortality and disability in advanced old age: the Newcastle 85+ study. J Clin Endocrinol Metab. 2016;101:4385–94.
5. Wang D, Li D, Guo X, et al. Effects of sex, age, sampling time, and season on thyroid-stimulating hormone concentrations: a retrospective study. Biochem Biophys Res Commun. 2018;506:450–4.

6. Surks MI, Hollowell JG. Age-specific distribution of serum thyrotropin and antithyroid antibodies in the US population: implications for the prevalence of subclinical hypothyroidism. J Clin Endocrinol Metab. 2007;92:4575–82.

7. Lewis GF, Alessi CA, Imperial JG, Refetoff S. Low serum free thyroxine index in ambulating elderly is due to a resetting of the threshold of thyrotropin feedback suppression. J Clin Endocrinol Metab. 1991;73:843–9.

8. Jansen SW, Akintola AA, Roelfsema F, et al. Human longevity is characterised by high thyroid stimulating hormone secretion without altered energy metabolism. Sci Rep. 2015;5:11525.

9. Ceresini G, Marina M, Lauretani F, et al. Relationship between circulating thyroid-stimulating hormone, free thyroxine, and free triiodothyronine concentrations and 9-year mortality in euthyroid elderly adults. J Am Geriatr Soc. 2016;64:553–60.

10. Gussekloo J, van Exel E, de Craen AJ, Meinders AE, Frölich M, Westendorp RG. Thyroid status, disability and cognitive function, and survival in old age. JAMA. 2004;292:2591–9.

11. Yeap BB, Alfonso H, Hankey GJ, et al. Higher free thyroxine levels are associated with all-cause mortality in euthyroid older men: the health in men study. Eur J Endocrinol. 2013;169:401–8.

12. Waring AC, Arnold AM, Newman AB, Bùzková P, Hirsch C, Cappola AR. Longitudinal changes in thyroid function in the oldest old and survival: the cardiovascular health study all-stars study. J Clin Endocrinol Metab. 2012;97:3944–50.

13. Golledge J, Hankey GJ, Almeida OP, Flicker L, Norman PE, Yeap BB. Plasma free thyroxine in the upper quartile is associated with an increased incidence of major cardiovascular events in older men that do not have thyroid dysfunction according to conventional criteria. Int J Cardiol. 2018;254:316–21.

14. Nanchen D, Gussekloo J, Westendorp RG, et al. Subclinical thyroid dysfunction and the risk of heart failure in older persons at high cardiovascular risk. J Clin Endocrinol Metab. 2012;97:852–61.

15. Yeap BB, Alfonso H, Chubb SA, et al. Higher free thyroxine levels are associated with frailty in older men: the health in men study. Clin Endocrinol (Oxf). 2012;76:741–8.

16. Yeap BB, Alfonso H, Chubb SA, et al. Higher free thyroxine levels predict increased incidence of dementia in older men: the health in men study. J Clin Endocrinol Metab. 2012;97:E2230–7.

17. Eskelinen SI, Vahlberg TJ, Isoaho RE, Löppönen MK, Kivelä SL, Irjala KM. Associations of thyroid-stimulating hormone and free thyroxine concentrations with health and life satisfaction in elderly adults. Endocr Pract. 2007;13:451–7.

18. Simonsick EM, Chia CW, Mammen JS, Egan JM, Ferrucci L. Free thyroxine and functional mobility, fitness, and fatigue in euthyroid older men and women in the Baltimore Longitudinal Study of Aging. J Gerontol A Biol Sci Med Sci. 2016;71:961–7.

19. Mingote E, Meroño T, Rujelman R, et al. High TSH and low T4 as prognostic markers in older patients. Hormones (Athens). 2012;11:350–5.

20. Volpato S, Guralnik JM, Fried LP, Remaley AT, Cappola AR, Launer LJ. Serum thyroxine level and cognitive decline in euthyroid older women. Neurology. 2002;58:1055–61.

21. Ochs N, Auer R, Bauer DC, et al. Meta-analysis: subclinical thyroid dysfunction and the risk for coronary heart disease and mortality. Ann Intern Med. 2008;148:832–45.

22. Razvi S, Shakoor A, Vanderpump M, Weaver JU, Pearce SH. The influence of age on the relationship between subclinical hypothyroidism and ischemic heart disease: a metaanalysis. J Clin Endocrinol Metab. 2008;93:2998–3007.

23. Stott DJ, Gussekloo J, Kearney PM, et al. Study protocol; thyroid hormone replacement for untreated older adults with subclinical hypothyroidism—a randomised placebo controlled trial (TRUST). BMC Endocr Disord. 2017;17:6.

24. Stott DJ, Rodondi N, Kearney PM, et al. Thyroid hormone therapy for older adults with subclinical hypothyroidism. N Engl J Med. 2017;376:2534–44.

25. Razvi S, Peeters R, Pearce SHS. Thyroid hormone therapy for subclinical hypothyroidism. JAMA. 2019;321:804.

26. de Montmollin M, Feller M, Beglinger S, et al. L-thyroxine therapy for older adults with subclinical hypothyroidism and hypothyroid symptoms: secondary analysis of a randomized trial. Ann Intern Med. 2020;172:709–16.

27. Gencer B, Moutzouri E, Blum MR, et al. The impact of levothyroxine on cardiac function in older adults with mild subclinical hypothyroidism: a randomized clinical trial. Am J Med. 2020;133:848–856.e5.

28. Gonzalez Rodriguez E, Stuber M, Del Giovane C, et al. Skeletal effects of levothyroxine for subclinical hypothyroidism in older adults: a TRUST randomized trial nested study. J Clin Endocrinol Metab. 2020;105:dgz058.

29. Mooijaart SP, Du Puy RS, Stott DJ, et al. Association between levothyroxine treatment and thyroid-related symptoms among adults aged 80 years and older with subclinical hypothyroidism. JAMA. 2019;322:1–11.

30. Parle J, Roberts L, Wilson S, et al. A randomized controlled trial of the effect of thyroxine replacement on cognitive function in community-living elderly subjects with subclinical hypothyroidism: the Birmingham Elderly Thyroid study. J Clin Endocrinol Metab. 2010;95:3623–32.

31. Jaeschke R, Guyatt G, Gerstein H, et al. Does treatment with L-thyroxine influence health status in middle-aged and older adults with subclinical hypothyroidism? J Gen Intern Med. 1996;11:744–9.

32. Feller M, Snel M, Moutzouri E, et al. Association of thyroid hormone therapy with quality of life and thyroid-related symptoms in patients with subclinical hypothyroidism: a systematic review and meta-analysis. JAMA. 2018;320:1349–59.

33. Blum MR, Gencer B, Adam L, et al. Impact of thyroid hormone therapy on atherosclerosis in the elderly with subclinical hypothyroidism: a randomized trial. J Clin Endocrinol Metab. 2018;103:2988–97.

34. Recker S, Voigtländer R, Viehmann A, et al. Thyroid related quality of life in elderly with subclinical hypothyroidism and improvement on levothyroxine is distinct from that in young patients (TSAGE). Horm Metab Res. 2019;51:568–74.

35. Moon JH, Han JW, Oh TJ, et al. Effect of increased levothyroxine dose on depressive mood in older adults undergoing thyroid hormone replacement therapy. Clin Endocrinol (Oxf). 2020;93:196–203.

36. Blum MR, Bauer DC, Collet TH, et al. Subclinical thyroid dysfunction and fracture risk: a meta-analysis. JAMA. 2015;313:2055–65.

37. Swedish Council on Health Technology Assessment. Osteoporosis—prevention, diagnosis and treatment: a systematic review [Internet]. Stockholm: Swedish Council on Health Technology Assessment (SBU); Oct 2003. SBU Yellow Report No. 165/1+2. Available at https://www.ncbi.nlm.nih.gov/books/NBK447989/. Accessed Jul 2020.

38. Ko YJ, Kim JY, Lee J, et al. Levothyroxine dose and fracture risk according to the osteoporosis status in elderly women. J Prev Med Public Health. 2014;47:36–46.

39. Turner MR, Camacho X, Fischer HD, et al. Levothyroxine dose and risk of fractures in older adults: nested case-control study. BMJ. 2011;342:d2238.

40. Mammen JS, McGready J, Oxman R, Chia CW, Ladenson PW, Simonsick EM. Thyroid hormone therapy and risk of thyrotoxicosis in community-resident older adults: findings from the Baltimore Longitudinal Study of Aging. Thyroid. 2015;25:979–86.

41. Thayakaran R, Adderley NJ, Sainsbury C, et al. Thyroid replacement therapy, thyroid stimulating hormone concentrations, and long term health outcomes in patients with hypothyroidism: longitudinal study. BMJ. 2019;366:l4892.

42. Wilkes S, Pearce S, Ryan V, Rapley T, Ingoe L, Razvi S. Study of Optimal Replacement of Thyroxine in the ElDerly (SORTED): protocol for a mixed methods feasibility study to assess the clinical utility of lower dose thyroxine in elderly hypothyroid patients: study protocol for a randomized controlled trial. Trials. 2013;14:83.

43. Razvi S, Ingoe L, Ryan V, Pearce SH, Wilkes S. Study of Optimal Replacement of Thyroxine in the Elderly (SORTED)—results from the feasibility randomised controlled trial. Thyroid Res. 2016;9:5.
44. Razvi S, Ryan V, Ingoe L, Pearce SH, Wilkes S. Age-related serum thyroid-stimulating hormone reference range in older patients treated with levothyroxine: a randomized controlled feasibility trial (SORTED 1). Eur Thyroid J. 2020;9:40–8.
45. Jonklaas J, Bianco AC, Bauer AJ, et al. Guidelines for the treatment of hypothyroidism: prepared by the American Thyroid Association task force on thyroid hormone replacement. Thyroid. 2014;24:1670–751.
46. Pearce SH, Brabant G, Duntas LH, et al. 2013 ETA guideline: management of subclinical hypothyroidism. Eur Thyroid J. 2013;2:215–28.
47. Cappola AR. The thyrotropin reference range should be changed in older patients. JAMA. 2020 (advance publication online, https://doi.org/10.1001/jama.2019.14728).

Levothyroxine and the Heart

Bernadette Biondi

Thyroid hormone deficiency has been associated with multiple changes in cardiovascular structure and function in recent studies. A strong relationship has been reported between overt and subclinical hypothyroidism with serum TSH ≥10 mIU/L and adverse cardiovascular outcomes, suggesting the necessity of replacement doses of Levothyroxine. The potential benefits of replacement therapy remain an active area of research in euthyroid patients with heart failure.

1 Introduction

Hypothyroidism is a common condition of thyroid hormone deficiency which can lead to increased cardiovascular mortality when untreated. Overt hypothyroidism is defined by thyroxine concentrations below the reference range and a serum thyrotropin (thyroid-stimulating hormone, TSH) measurement that is outside an appropriate reference range (typically between 0.4 and 4.0–4.5 mIU/L, defined in a population of subjects without thyroid disease) [1, 2]. Subclinical hypothyroidism occurs where there is elevation of TSH despite the level of free thyroxine (FT4) being within the normal reference range. Patients with a serum TSH ≥10 mIU/L have a severe form of subclinical hypothyroidism, whereas patients with subclinical hypothyroidism and TSH <10 mIU/L are described as having a "mild" form of this condition, according to European guidance [1]. This chapter considers the effects of hypothyroidism and levothyroxine (LT4) replacement therapy on the heart and cardiovascular system.

B. Biondi (✉)
Professor of Endocrinology and Internal Medicine, University of Naples Federico II, Naples, Italy
e-mail: bebiondi@unina.it

© The Author(s) 2021
G. J. Kahaly (ed.), *70 Years of Levothyroxine*,
https://doi.org/10.1007/978-3-030-63277-9_7

Table 1 Overview of observational studies of the associations between thyroid status and cardiovascular health that recruited at least 1000 subjects

Refs.	Cardiovascular outcome in patients with hypothyroidism
Population based (without known thyroid dysfunction and with/without CHD at baseline)	
[3–5]	No association between SCH or overt hypothyroidism and MACE
[6]	SCH and overt hypothyroidism associated with higher all-cause mortality and increased risk of MACE (but mortality was lower for TSH 5–10 mIU/L)
[7]	SCH increased risk of mortality in acute CHD
[8]	SCH associated with increased prevalence of CHD, and higher than expected rate of MACE
[9]	SCH increased the risk of all-cause and CV mortality
[10]	SCH increased risk of stroke in adults
[11]	SCH increased total and CHD mortality
[12]	Increased 10-year CVD risk score in people with SCH vs. euthyroid
Patients with or at risk of heart failure (HF)	
[13]	Higher TSH associated with more severe CHF presentation
[13, 14]	Higher TSH associated with adverse clinical outcomes in patients with HF
[15]	Hypothyroidism predicted adverse clinical outcomes, but the association was not independent and disappeared after adjustment for other covariates
[16]	Low FT3 associated with higher risk of developing HF after myocardial infarction
[17]	Hypothyroidism increased the 5-year risk of death in patients with LVEF <35%
[18]	TSH ≥10 mIU/L increased the risk of new-onset HF, increased LV mass, and decreased diastolic function in patients free of HF at baseline
[19]	SCH increased the risk of HF in older subjects at elevated CV risk

2 Overview of the Adverse Effects of Thyroid Dysfunction on the Heart

Many observational studies have evaluated cardiovascular function in people with hypothyroidism and Table 1 summarises the results of some large, recent studies [3–19]. The findings of these studies were variable, probably because of differences between populations in terms of the severity of hypothyroidism, the age of the patients, and the presence of comorbidities. Nevertheless, expert opinions reported a significant association between hypothyroidism with scrum TSH ≥10 mIU/L and adverse cardiovascular outcomes [20, 21]. A systematic review demonstrated multiple effects of subclinical hypothyroidism on the heart that were consistent with reduced diastolic or systolic cardiac left ventricular performance, and some of its key findings are summarised in Table 2 [21, 22]. In contrast, a meta-analysis found that the presence or absence of anti-thyroid peroxidase antibodies neither increases nor reduces the risk of adverse cardiovascular outcomes in people with subclinical hypothyroidism [23].

Table 2 Overview of the effects of subclinical hypothyroidism and levothyroxine replacement therapy on the heart, from a systematic review

	Left ventricular diastolic function			LV systolic function		Lipid profiles		
	A wave	E/A ratio	IRT	PEP	PEP/ ET	Total cholesterol	LDL-cholesterol	HDL-cholesterol
Effect of subclinical hypothyroidism	↑	↓ or ↔	↑	↑[a]	↑[a]	↑ or ↔	↑ or ↔	↑ or ↔
Effect of LT4 replacement	↓	↑	↑	–	↓	↓ or ↔	↓ or ↔	↔↑

Changes in parameters reflect those seen in most (not necessarily all) studies: ↑ = increased; ↓ = decreased; ↔ = variable effects

E/A early-to-late transmitral peak flow velocity ratio, *ET* ejection time, *IRT* isovolumic relaxation time, *LV* left ventricular, *PEP* pre-ejection period. Compiled from information presented in Refs. [21, 22]

[a]Usually increased when measured using Doppler ultrasound (usually no effect when measured using Weissler's method)

Results of studies that evaluated the relationships between thyroid status and the lipid profile have also been variable although there is some evidence that more severe increases in TSH are associated with a more adverse change in the lipid profile [22]. Effects of the hypothyroid state on "non-traditional" cardiovascular risk factors (e.g. markers of haemostasis or systemic inflammation) were variable although there was some support for a possible action of hypothyroidism in exacerbating atherosclerosis [22].

The association of hypothyroidism with adverse cardiovascular outcomes appears to be stronger and most consistent for people with heart failure [24–26]. A recent (2019) meta-analysis of 14 studies (21,221 patients) found a significant association between hypothyroidism (including the subclinical form) and major prognostic outcomes associated with heart failure, such as cardiac death and/or hospitalisation [27]. A pooled analysis of prospective cohort studies showed that the risk of heart failure events (any physician-diagnosed acute heart failure event, or hospitalization or death related to heart failure) increased as the level of TSH increased above a euthyroid range defined as a TSH level of 0.45–4.49 mIU/L [28]. The hazard ratio (HR) for heart failure events for TSH 7–9.9 mIU/L vs. the euthyroid state was 1.65 (95%CI 0.84–3.23). TSH levels associated with hyperthyroidism also increased the risk of heart failure events in this analysis. Elsewhere, 12 years of prospective follow-up of 3,044 elderly (age ≥65 years) subjects with subclinical hypothyroidism showed that a TSH level >10 mIU/L was associated with an almost doubled risk of developing new heart failure HR 1.88; 95%CI 10.5–3.34) [18]. On the other hand, cardiovascular diseases such as heart failure may themselves lead to an altered thyroid function [29]. Low circulating T3 levels are a common finding in patients with heart failure and contribute to adverse outcomes in this condition [25].

3   Effects of Levothyroxine Replacement Therapy on the Cardiovascular System

3.1   Effects on ECG Parameters

Hypothyroid patients have abnormal heart rate variability compared with euthyroid controls, which can be corrected by an adequate LT4 replacement therapy [30]. Ambulatory ECG recording showed that long-term LT4 replacement appears to avoid the bradyarrhythmias commonly associated with hypothyroidism [31]. Moreover, LT4 treatment may reduce QT interval dispersion in patients with subclinical hypothyroidism, reducing the risk of malignant cardiac arrhythmias [32].

3.2   Effects of L-Thyroxine on Cardiovascular Structure and Function

Subclinical hypothyroidism appears to represent a mild form of thyroid failure that displays early signs of the cardiovascular dysfunction associated with hypothyroidism [33, 34]. The impairment in systolic and/or diastolic performance observed in patients with subclinical hypothyroidism, compared with healthy controls, has been shown to reverse during treatment with LT4 for periods of up to 1 year (Table 2) [21]. Such effects have been observed in young adults but not in elderly subjects in some randomized trials [35–37].

An overview of these and other studies in populations with subclinical hypothyroidism are summarised in Table 3 [32, 35–51]. Markers of atherosclerosis or arterial stiffness improved in some studies [39, 52]. A further cross-sectional analysis demonstrated an improvement in atrial volume [53]. Another randomised trial showed that treatment with LT4 improved cholesterol levels in people with subclinical hypothyroidism [39]. In addition, patients with mild subclinical hypothyroidism without associated cardiovascular risk factors have a coronary endothelial dysfunction that appears in response to a physiological stimulus [54]. A meta-analysis found an improved lipid profile and reduced carotid intima-media thickness (a marker of the overall burden of atherosclerosis) in patients with subclinical hypothyroidism [38]. Finally, treatment with LT4 may reduce cardiovascular risk in patients with diabetes: increased prevalence of thyroid dysfunction in patients with diabetes (and *vice versa*) suggests that there may be pathogenetic links between these conditions [55].

Thus, clinical evidence has associated overt and severe subclinical hypothyroidism with indices of increased cardiovascular risk, including dyslipidaemia, impaired cardiac function (especially during diastole) and impaired vascular function [56]. Evidence of potentially beneficial cardiovascular effects of LT4 replacement therapy on these parameters has led some experts to propose intervention with LT4 in patients with mild subclinical hypothyroidism and elevated cardiovascular risk factors. However, until more reliable evidence is available from randomised,

Table 3 Clinical evaluations of the cardiovascular effects of levothyroxine substitution in people with subclinical hypothyroidism

Ref.	Design/dur. of LT4	N	Précis of main findings
(a)	*Effects of LT4 replacement therapy on lipid profiles and markers of atherosclerosis*		
[38]	MA up to 1 year	543	LT4 replacement improved total and LDL-C and reduced markers of vascular disease (carotid atherosclerosis and arterial stiffness
[39]	RCT 6 months	49	Patients with SCH had higher cholesterol, LDL-C and ApoB vs. 33 euthyroid controls (LDL-C was proportional to the TSH level). Randomisation to LT4 resulted in reduced cholesterol and LDL-C, with no change in Lp(a); there were no significant changes on placebo.
[40]	O, 7 months	30	Blood pressure and augmentation index (measure of arterial stiffness) decreased on LT4 therapy; reduced augmentation index was associated with reduced LDL-C
[41]	O, 6 months	33	In patients with CHD, LT4 treatment improved the lipid profile in patients with shorter duration of CHD, lower BMI and higher cholesterol at baseline.
(b)	*Effects of LT4 replacement therapy on cardiac function*		
[37]	RCT, 18 months	185	No significant difference for LT4 vs. placebo for changes in LV ejection fraction, E/E' ratio or other parameters relating to diastolic functional; no significant interactions relating to gender, baseline TSH, pre-existing HF, and treatment duration
[35]	RCT, 6 months	42	Increased early diastolic velocity and ratio of early/late diastolic velocities and reduced isovolumetric relaxation time was observed after 6 months of LT4; no change was seen in untreated patients
[36]	RCT, 1 year	20	LT4 associated with reversal of impairments (vs. euthyroid controls) in pre-ejection/ejection time ratio, peak A, isovolumic relaxation time, cyclic variation index (myocardial viability); no significant changes on placebo.
[42]	O, 6 months	30	Significant increase in indices of LV contractility (ejection fraction, fractional shortening, myocardial performance index) and end diastolic LV diameter in children; no change in LV end systolic volume or diastolic function (*E/E'* ratio).
[43]	O, 6 months[a]	31	Adverse changes in parameters of systolic and diastolic function in SCH (compared with 32 euthyroid control children) were partially reversed on LT4 replacement therapy.
[44]	O, 5 months[a]	54	Parameters relating to systolic and diastolic function were within normal range in newly diagnosed SCH patients but were significantly adverse compared with 30 euthyroid controls; LT4 replacement partially reversed these changes.
[45]	O, 12 months	26	Impairments (vs. 13 healthy controls) in systolic and diastolic cardiac function parameters (LV ejection fraction, diastolic relaxation, compliance to ventricular filling) reversed after LT4 therapy.

(continued)

Table 3 (continued)

Ref.	Design/dur. of LT4	N	Précis of main findings
[46]	O, 6 months[a]	53	Multiple indices of systolic/diastolic right ventricular function were impaired vs. 25 euthyroid controls; LT4 associated with improved isovolumic acceleration (no change in systolic wave velocity, early/late velocity or myocardial precontraction times.
[32]	O, 16 weeks	16	Treatment with LT4 reduced the QT interval of the ECG, and its temporal dispersion (QT interval dispersion was proportional to the TSH level).
(c) Effects of LT4 replacement therapy on clinical outcomes			
[47]	RT, mean 38 months	257	LT4 replacement for ≥180 days (vs. <180 days) predicted significantly lower risk of acute coronary syndromes or stroke, but no effect on peripheral vascular disease in patients with diabetic neuropathy (average follow-up 38 months).
[48]	RT, median 6 years	162,369	Increased risk (HR [95%CI]) at TSH >10 vs. 2–2.5 mIU/L of IHD (1.18 [1.02–1.38], $p = 0.03$), HF (1.42 [1.21–1.67], $p < 0.001$), or mortality (2.21 [2.07–2.36] $p < 0.001$) in an LT4-treated cohort (97% received LT4 during follow-up)
[49]	RCT, mean 5.6 years	1192	No significant difference for LT4 vs. no LT4 treatment (adjusted IRR [95%CI]) for risk of all-cause death (1.17 [0.90–1.52), MACE (1.08 [0.80–1.45]), or hospital admission (0.94 [0.71–1.24]) in patients with CHD.
[50]	RCT, mean 5.0 years	12,212	No significant effect of LT4 vs. no LT4 on IRR [95%CI] for MI (1.08 [0.81–1.44]), CV death (1.02 [0.83–1.25]), all-cause death (1.03 [0.90–1.19]); suggestion of benefit for all-cause death in patients aged <65 years (0.63 [0.40–0.99]).
[51]	RCT, mean 7.6 years	4735	Fewer IHD events (HR [95%CI]) with LT4 treatment in younger (40–70 years) patients (0.61 [0.39–0.95]) but not in older (≥70 years) patients (HR 0.99 [0.59–1.33]) in the primary care setting.

Diagnoses of subclinical hypothyroidism are as described in source publications according to clinical guidance at the time and have not been reviewed against current guidance

Abbreviations for study designs: *DB* double blind, *MA* meta-analysis (individual studies included in this analysis are omitted here for conciseness), *O* observational/cohort study, *R* randomised, *RT* retrospective. Other abbreviations: *BMI* body mass index, *CHD* coronary heart disease, *HF* heart failure, *IHD* ischaemic heart disease, *IRR* incidence rate ratio, *LV* left ventricular, *MACE* major adverse cardiac events, *ACH* subclinical hypothyroidism, *TSH* thyroid-stimulating hormone (thyrotropin)

[a]Months with euthyroid function established on LT4 replacement therapy

controlled trials, intervention with LT4 should be considered on an individual, case-by-case basis, balancing the patient's potential for progressive thyroid failure with the need to protect the cardiovascular system [56].

An increase in left ventricular mass with a consequent diastolic dysfunction can be observed during long-term therapy with TSH-suppressive doses of LT4 [57, 58]. The addition of a β-blocker can ameliorate the potentially adverse effects of prolonged TSH suppression and be useful in patients with high-risk differentiated thyroid cancer [58]. The role of LT4 in the management of thyroid cancer is discussed in chapter, "Levothyroxine and Cancer" of this book.

3.3 Effects of LT4 on Major Adverse Cardiovascular Events

So far, only retrospective studies have evaluated the effects of LT4 treatment on cardiac endpoints in patients with subclinical hypothyroidism (Table 3c). The results of these studies, however, are variable. Two studies showed no significant effects of LT4 replacement on the risk of myocardial infarction, or on cardiovascular and all cause death [49, 50]. Intriguingly, there was a suggestion of a greater potential for cardiovascular benefit of LT4 therapy in younger than in older patients [51, 52]. A smaller study suggested some cardiovascular benefit for a longer rather than a shorter duration of LT4 treatment [47].

A large database analysis in a population with hypothyroidism, of whom 97% received LT4 during a median follow-up of 6 years, showed that treatment with LT4 *per se* was insufficient to protect the cardiovascular system if TSH was not normalised [48]. Specifically, under-treatment with LT4 (TSH >10 mIU/L) in this study was associated with increased risk of ischaemic heart disease (HR 1.18 [1.02–1.38], $p = 0.03$), heart failure (HR 1.42 [1.21–1.67], $p < 0.001$), or death (HR 2.21 [2.07–2.36], $p < 0.001$), compared with euthyroid subjects (TSH 2–2.5 mIU/L). A further, register-based study showed that every 6 months of elevated TSH was associated with increased risk of mortality in LT4-treated individuals, with identical risks (HR 1.05 [1.03–1.08], $p < 0.0001$) for TSH >4 IU/L or TSH >10 IU/L, compared with euthyroid controls (this study is not shown in Table 3, as it did not report cardiovascular outcomes) [59].

Treatment with LT4 for more than 1 year reduced the risk of developing CHD, compared with no LT4 treatment, in a large retrospective analysis from Taiwan [60]. The effect of LT4 therapy on clinical outcomes was also measured in a retrospective study on 12,283 patients with atrial fibrillation [61]. The adjusted risk of mortality was lower in women treated with LT4 (hazard ratio [HR] 0.78 [95%CI 0.68–0.91]), but not men (HR 0.87 [95%CI 0.69–1.10]) compared to those untreated. There was no significant effect of LT4 treatment on rates of myocardial infarction, stroke, or heart failure in this study. A large ($N = 87,902$) retrospective study saw no difference in cardiovascular outcomes between patients receiving a branded or generic preparation of LT4 [62].

3.4 Effects of LT4 in Patients with Heart Failure

A retrospective analysis of a large database of patients with heart failure from Denmark ($N = 224,670$) compared outcomes in non-users of LT4 and in 6,560 patients using LT4 at the start of the analysis, and in 9007 who subsequently received LT4 therapy [63]. Both groups of LT4 users were at increased risk of all-cause death, cardiovascular death, or MACE, compared with non-users. However, the risk of myocardial infarction was increased in patients already taking LT4 at baseline but reduced in patients who started LT4 during the follow-up period.

Large, randomized clinical trials of LT4 replacement therapy powered for determination of effects on clinical outcomes are lacking in populations of euthyroid subjects with heart failure and hypothyroidism. A placebo-controlled evaluation of LT4 treatment in 20 subjects with cardiac insufficiency secondary to idiopathic dilated cardiomyopathy demonstrated improvements in multiple measures of cardiac function, including LV ejection fraction, cardiac output, LV diastolic dimensions, systemic vascular resistance, and functional capacity [64, 65]. Another small ($N = 28$) study involved randomization of patients with severe symptoms of heart failure (New York Heart Association class III–IV) to LT4 supplementation or to no treatment for 1 month [66]. Significant improvements were seen in LV ejection fraction and isovolumic relaxation time in the LT4 group. An uncontrolled evaluation of LT4 in 10 patients with severe LV systolic dysfunction and cardiogenic shock demonstrated significant improvements in cardiac index, pulmonary capillary wedge pressure, and mean arterial blood pressure at times up to 36 h after treatment [67]. LT4 treatment also contributed to stabilization of the condition of 9/10 of these patients, allowing for surgical intervention (heart transplant or insertion of a mechanical device to assist the heart).

Administration of T3 in patients with heart failure has also been demonstrated to improve cardiac performance in patients with severe heart failure, in some [68, 69] but not all [70] studies. Although current guidance for the management of thyroid dysfunction (see chapter, "Pharmacodynamic and Therapeutic Actions of Levothyroxine") does not support the therapeutic use of preparations of T3, these findings are consistent with a role for thyroid dysfunction within the pathophysiology of heart failure, and with the importance of the low T3 syndrome in this setting [25]. The therapeutic use of T3 in patients with heart failure remains within the research domain, for now, and further clinical studies are needed in this area.

4 Conclusions

Hypothyroidism, including the severe form of subclinical hypothyroidism in which TSH is ≥ 10 mIU/L, has been associated with multiple negative changes in the structure and function of cardiovascular tissues and adverse cardiovascular outcomes. Some studies have shown that intervention with LT4 to correct hypothyroidism can result in a reduced risk of MACE although the results of studies are conflicting. Randomized clinical trials are needed and yet problematic in patients with overt hypothyroidism because management guidelines clearly state that all patients with this condition must be treated with LT4.

A potential role for LT4 therapy remains an active area of research in patients with subclinical hypothyroidism. It is particularly important to correct hypothyroidism and the more severe form of subclinical hypothyroidism in these patients [20, 21, 25]. Elderly patients with hypothyroidism may be especially challenging to manage, as they are more likely than younger patients to present with one or more cardiovascular comorbidities. For all patients, careful tailoring of the LT4 dose in hypothyroid patients should be performed to ovoid over-treatment and possible adverse effects on the cardiovascular system.

References

1. Pearce SH, Brabant G, Duntas LH, et al. 2013 ETA guideline: management of subclinical hypothyroidism. Eur Thyroid J. 2013;2:215–28.
2. Jonklaas J, Bianco AC, Bauer AJ, et al. Guidelines for the treatment of hypothyroidism: prepared by the American thyroid association task force on thyroid hormone replacement. Thyroid. 2014;24:1670–751.
3. Tohidi M, Derakhshan A, Akbarpour S, et al. Thyroid dysfunction states and incident cardiovascular events: the Tehran Thyroid Study. Horm Metab Res. 2018;50:37–43.
4. Martin SS, Daya N, Lutsey PL, et al. Thyroid function, cardiovascular risk factors, and incident atherosclerotic cardiovascular disease: the Atherosclerosis Risk in Communities (ARIC) Study. J Clin Endocrinol Metab. 2017;102:3306–15.
5. Zhao JV, Schooling CM. Thyroid function and ischemic heart disease: a Mendelian randomization study. Sci Rep. 2017;7:8515.
6. Selmer C, Olesen JB, Hansen ML, et al. Subclinical and overt thyroid dysfunction and risk of all-cause mortality and cardiovascular events: a large population study. J Clin Endocrinol Metab. 2014;99:2372–82.
7. Molinaro S, Iervasi G, Lorenzoni V, et al. Persistence of mortality risk in patients with acute cardiac diseases and mild thyroid dysfunction. Am J Med Sci. 2012;34:65–70.
8. Walsh JP, Bremner AP, Bulsara MK, et al. Subclinical thyroid dysfunction as a risk factor for cardiovascular disease. Arch Intern Med. 2005;165:2467–72.
9. Tseng FY, Lin WY, Lin CC, et al. Subclinical hypothyroidism is associated with increased risk for all-cause and cardiovascular mortality in adults. J Am Coll Cardiol. 2012;60:730–7.
10. Chaker L, Baumgartner C, den Elzen WP, et al. Subclinical hypothyroidism and the risk of stroke events and fatal stroke: an individual participant data analysis. J Clin Endocrinol Metab. 2015;100:2181–91.
11. Collet TH, Gussekloo J, Bauer DC, et al. Subclinical hyperthyroidism and the risk of coronary heart disease and mortality. Arch Intern Med. 2012;172:799–809.
12. Lim HJ, Ahn SH, Hong S, Suh YJ. The relationship between subclinical thyroid disease and cardiovascular disease risk score in Koreans. J Korean Med Sci. 2017;32:1626–32.
13. Kannan L, Shaw PA, Morley MP, et al. Thyroid dysfunction in heart failure and cardiovascular outcomes. Circ Heart Fail. 2018;11:e005266.
14. Chen S, Shauer A, Zwas DR, Lotan C, Keren A, Gotsman I. The effect of thyroid function on clinical outcome in patients with heart failure. Eur J Heart Fail. 2014;16:217–26.
15. Perez AC, Jhund PS, Stott DJ, et al. Thyroid-stimulating hormone and clinical outcomes: the CORONA trial (controlled rosuvastatin multinational study in heart failure). JACC Heart Fail. 2014;2:35–40.
16. Kang MG, Hahm JR, Kim KH, et al. Prognostic value of total triiodothyronine and free thyroxine levels for the heart failure in patients with acute myocardial infarction. Korean J Intern Med. 2018;33:512–21.
17. Mitchell JE, Hellkamp AS, Mark DB, et al. Thyroid function in heart failure and impact on mortality. JACC Heart Fail. 2013;1:48–55.

18. Rodondi N, Bauer DC, Cappola AR, et al. Subclinical thyroid dysfunction, cardiac function, and the risk of heart failure. The Cardiovascular Health Study. J Am Coll Cardiol. 2008;52:1152–9.
19. Nanchen D, Gussekloo J, Westendorp RG, et al. Subclinical thyroid dysfunction and the risk of heart failure in older persons at high cardiovascular risk. J Clin Endocrinol Metab. 2012;97:852–61.
20. Cooper DS, Biondi B. Subclinical thyroid disease. Lancet. 2012;379:1142–54.
21. Biondi B, Cappola AR, Cooper DS. Subclinical hypothyroidism: a review. JAMA. 2019;322:153–60.
22. Biondi B, Cooper DS. The clinical significance of subclinical thyroid dysfunction. Endocr Rev. 2008;29:76–131.
23. Collet TH, Bauer DC, Cappola AR, et al. Thyroid antibody status, subclinical hypothyroidism, and the risk of coronary heart disease: an individual participant data analysis. J Clin Endocrinol Metab. 2014;99:3353–62.
24. Biondi B. Mechanisms in endocrinology: heart failure and thyroid dysfunction. Eur J Endocrinol. 2012;167:609–18.
25. Biondi B. The management of thyroid abnormalities in chronic heart failure. Heart Fail Clin. 2019;15:393–8.
26. Vargas-Uricoechea H, Bonelo-Perdomo A. Thyroid dysfunction and heart failure: mechanisms and associations. Curr Heart Fail Rep. 2017;14:48–58.
27. Yang G, Wang Y, Ma A, Wang T. Subclinical thyroid dysfunction is associated with adverse prognosis in heart failure patients with reduced ejection fraction. BMC Cardiovasc Disord. 2019;19:83.
28. Gencer B, Collet TH, Virgini V, et al. Subclinical thyroid dysfunction and the risk of heart failure events: an individual participant data analysis from 6 prospective cohorts. Circulation. 2012;126:1040–9.
29. Danzi S, Klein I. Thyroid abnormalities in heart failure. Heart Fail Clin. 2020;16:1–9.
30. Xing H, Shen Y, Chen H, Wang Y, Shen W. Heart rate variability and its response to thyroxine replacement therapy in patients with hypothyroidism. Chin Med J (Engl). 2001;114:906–8.
31. Hylander B, Kennebäck G, Rosenqvist U, Edhag O. Long-term ECG recordings in thyroxine-substituted hypothyroid subjects. Acta Med Scand. 1987;222:429–32.
32. Unal O, Erturk E, Ozkan H, et al. Effect of levothyroxine treatment on QT dispersion in patients with subclinical hypothyroidism. Endocr Pract. 2007;13:711–5.
33. Biondi B, Palmieri EA, Lombardi G, Fazio S. Subclinical hypothyroidism and cardiac function. Thyroid. 2002;12:505–10.
34. Biondi B, Palmieri EA, Lombardi G, Fazio S. Effects of subclinical thyroid dysfunction on the heart. Ann Intern Med. 2002;137:904–14.
35. Franzoni F, Galetta F, Fallahi P, et al. Effect of L-thyroxine treatment on left ventricular function in subclinical hypothyroidism. Biomed Pharmacother. 2006;60:431–6.
36. Monzani F, Di Bello V, Caraccio N, et al. Effect of levothyroxine on cardiac function and structure in subclinical hypothyroidism: a double blind, placebo-controlled study. J Clin Endocrinol Metab. 2001;86:1110–5.
37. Gencer B, Moutzouri E, Blum MR, et al. The impact of levothyroxine on cardiac function in older adults with mild subclinical hypothyroidism: a randomized clinical trial. Am J Med. 2020;133:848–56.e5.
38. Aziz M, Kandimalla Y, Machavarapu A, et al. Effect of thyroxin treatment on carotid intima-media thickness (CIMT) reduction in patients with subclinical hypothyroidism (sch): a meta-analysis of clinical trials. J Atheroscler Thromb. 2017;24:643–59.
39. Caraccio N, Ferrannini E, Monzani F. Lipoprotein profile in subclinical hypothyroidism: response to levothyroxine replacement, a randomized placebo-controlled study. J Clin Endocrinol Metab. 2002;87:1533–8.
40. Peleg RK, Efrati S, Benbassat C, Fygenzo M, Golik A. The effect of levothyroxine on arterial stiffness and lipid profile in patients with subclinical hypothyroidism. Thyroid. 2008;18:825–30.

41. Fadeyev VV, Sytch J, Kalashnikov V, Rojtman A, Syrkin A, Melnichenko G. Levothyroxine replacement therapy in patients with subclinical hypothyroidism and coronary artery disease. Endocr Pract. 2006;12:5–17.
42. Banu Rupani N, Alijanpour M, Babazadeh K, Hajian-Tilaki K, Moadabdoost F. Effect of levothyroxine on cardiac function in children with subclinical hypothyroidism: a quasi-experimental study. Caspian J Intern Med. 2019;10:332–8.
43. Çatli G, Kir M, Anik A, Yilmaz N, Böber E, Abaci A. The effect of L-thyroxine treatment on left ventricular functions in children with subclinical hypothyroidism. Arch Dis Child. 2015;100:130–7.
44. Nakova VV, Krstevska B, Kostovska ES, Vaskova O, Ismail LG. The effect of levothyroxine treatment on left ventricular function in subclinical hypothyroidism. Arch Endocrinol Metab. 2018;62:392–8.
45. Mariotti S, Zoncu S, Pigliaru F, et al. Cardiac effects of L-thyroxine administration in borderline hypothyroidism. Int J Cardiol. 2008;126:190–5.
46. Turhan S, Tulunay C, Ozduman Cin M, et al. Effects of thyroxine therapy on right ventricular systolic and diastolic function in patients with subclinical hypothyroidism: a study by pulsed wave tissue Doppler imaging. J Clin Endocrinol Metab. 2006;91:3490–3.
47. Seo C, Kim S, Lee M, Cha MU, et al. Thyroid hormone replacement reduces the risk of cardiovascular diseases in diabetic nephropathy patients with subclinical hypothyroidism. Endocr Pract. 2018;24:265–72.
48. Thayakaran R, Adderley NJ, Sainsbury C, et al. Thyroid replacement therapy, thyroid stimulating hormone concentrations, and long term health outcomes in patients with hypothyroidism: longitudinal study. BMJ. 2019;366:l4892.
49. Andersen MN, Olsen AS, Madsen JC, et al. Long-term outcome in levothyroxine treated patients with subclinical hypothyroidism and concomitant heart disease. J Clin Endocrinol Metab. 2016;101:4170–7.
50. Andersen MN, Olsen AM, Madsen JC, et al. Levothyroxine substitution in patients with subclinical hypothyroidism and the risk of myocardial infarction and mortality. PLoS One. 2015;10:e0129793.
51. Razvi S, Weaver JU, Butler TJ, Pearce SH. Levothyroxine treatment of subclinical hypothyroidism, fatal and nonfatal cardiovascular events, and mortality. Arch Intern Med. 2012;172: 811–7.
52. del Busto-Mesa A, Cabrera-Rego JO, Carrero-Fernández L, et al. Changes in arterial stiffness, carotid intima-media thickness, and epicardial fat after L-thyroxine replacement therapy in hypothyroidism. Endocrinol Nutr. 2015;62:270–6.
53. Dereli S, Bayramoğlu A, Özer N, Kaya A, Özbilen M. Evaluation of left atrial volume and functions by real time three-dimensional echocardiography in patients with subclinical hypothyroidism before and after levothyroxine therapy. Echocardiography. 2019;36:916–23.
54. Biondi B, Galderisi M, Pagano L, et al. Endothelial-mediated coronary flow reserve in patients with mild thyroid hormone deficiency. Eur J Endocrinol. 2009;161:323–9.
55. Biondi B, Kahaly GJ, Robertson RP. Thyroid dysfunction and diabetes mellitus: two closely associated disorders. Endocr Rev. 2019;40:789–824.
56. Palmieri EA, Fazio S, Lombardi G, Biondi B. Subclinical hypothyroidism and cardiovascular risk: a reason to treat? Treat Endocrinol. 2004;3:233–44.
57. Mercuro G, Panzuto MG, Bina A, Leo M, Cabula R, Petrini L. Cardiac function, physical exercise capacity, and quality of life during long-term thyrotropin-suppressive therapy with levothyroxine: effect of individual dose tailoring. J Clin Endocrinol Metab. 2000;85: 159–64.
58. Fazio S, Biondi B, Carella C, et al. Diastolic dysfunction in patients on thyroid-stimulating hormone suppressive therapy with levothyroxine: beneficial effect of beta-blockade. J Clin Endocrinol Metab. 1995;80:2222–6.
59. Lillevang-Johansen M, Abrahamsen B, Jørgensen HL, Brix TH, Hegedüs L. Over- and under-treatment of hypothyroidism is associated with excess mortality: a register-based cohort study. Thyroid. 2018;28:566–74.

60. Chen WH, Chen YK, Lin CL, Yeh JH, Kao CH. Hashimoto's thyroiditis, risk of coronary heart disease, and L-thyroxine treatment: a nationwide cohort study. J Clin Endocrinol Metab. 2015;100:109–14.
61. Wändell P, Carlsson AC, Holzmann MJ, Ärnlöv J, Sundquist J, Sundquist K. Comparison of mortality and nonfatal cardiovascular events in adults with atrial fibrillation with versus without levothyroxine treatment. Am J Cardiol. 2017;120:1974–9.
62. Smallridge RC, Sangaralingham LR, Mwangi R, Kusumoto F, Van Houten H, Bernet V. Comparison of incident cardiovascular event rates between generic and brand l-thyroxine for the treatment of hypothyroidism. Mayo Clin Proc. 2019;94:1190–8.
63. Einfeldt MN. Olsen AS1, Kristensen SL, et al. long-term outcome in patients with heart failure treated with levothyroxine: an observational nationwide cohort study. J Clin Endocrinol Metab. 2019;104:1725–34.
64. Moruzzi P, Doria E, Agostoni PG, Capacchione V, Sganzerla P. Usefulness of L-thyroxine to improve cardiac and exercise performance in idiopathic dilated cardiomyopathy. Am J Cardiol. 1994;73:374–8.
65. Moruzzi P, Doria E, Agostoni PG. Medium-term effectiveness of L-thyroxine treatment in idiopathic dilated cardiomyopathy. Am J Med. 1996;101:461–7.
66. Lu X, Huang J, Zhang X, et al. Effects of thyroxine on cardiac function and lymphocyte beta-adrenoceptors in patients with chronic congestive heart failure. Chin Med J (Engl). 2003;116:1697–700.
67. Malik FS, Mehra MR, Uber PA, Park MH, Scott RL, Van Meter CH. Intravenous thyroid hormone supplementation in heart failure with cardiogenic shock. J Card Fail. 1999;5:31–7.
68. Pingitore A, Iervasi G. Triiodothyronine (T3) effects on cardiovascular system in patients with heart failure. Recent Pat Cardiovasc Drug Discov. 2008;3:19–27.
69. Hamilton MA, Stevenson LW, Fonarow GC, et al. Safety and hemodynamic effects of intravenous triiodothyronine in advanced congestive heart failure. Am J Cardiol. 1998;81:443–7.
70. Holmager P, Schmidt U, Mark P, et al. Long-term L-Triiodothyronine (T3) treatment in stable systolic heart failure patients: a randomised, double-blind, cross-over, placebo-controlled intervention study. Clin Endocrinol (Oxf). 2015;83:931–7.

Levothyroxine and Bone

Weiping Teng

Thyroid hormones play an important role in the development of the skeleton in children, and in maintaining bone mineral content in adults. Hyperthyroidism is associated with loss of bone mineral content, with increased risk of fractures. This has raised concerns that treatment (especially over treatment) with levothyroxine (LT4) might mimic these adverse effects on the skeleton. Clinical data on the effects of LT4 administration on bone are conflicting. In general, the use of LT4 to maintain euthyroid levels of thyroid hormones in patients with hypothyroidism, or even the use of thyrotropin-suppressive therapy following removal of thyroid tumours, does not appear to carry a substantial risk of osteoporosis or fractures. Nevertheless, a cautious approach to avoid over treatment is recommended, especially in patients with or at risk of developing osteoporosis.

1 Overview of the Effects of Thyroid Hormones on the Skeleton

Thyroid hormones (principally triiodothyronine, derived from naturally produced thyroxine or exogenously administered levothyroxine [LT4]) are essential for the normal development of the skeleton [1, 2]. Untreated congenital hypothyroidism, where there is a profound lack of thyroid function from birth, is associated with delayed development of the skeleton, impaired development of epiphyseal growth plates, short stature (dwarfism), reduced mineralisation of bones, scoliosis and congenital hip displacement, among other complications [1, 2]. Reduced bone turnover

W. Teng (✉)
First Hospital of China Medical University, Shenyang, China

Institute of Endocrinology, China Medical University, Shenyang, China
e-mail: twp@vip.163.com

© The Author(s) 2021
G. J. Kahaly (ed.), *70 Years of Levothyroxine*,
https://doi.org/10.1007/978-3-030-63277-9_8

in adults with hypothyroidism may result in increased bone mineralisation and mass, but such changes are slow to develop and this phenomenon has not been well studied clinically [2]. Hypothyroidism is not strongly associated with fractures [3, 4] although one meta-analysis described such a relationship that was apparently independently of changes in bone mineral density (BMD).

Hyperthyroidism increases the rate of turnover of bone, with a net loss of bone mineralisation; accordingly, suboptimally managed hyperthyroidism can be a cause of osteoporosis and increased fracture risk [1, 2]. Restoration of euthyroid status reverses the loss of bone mineral content and also ameliorates the excess fracture risk in patients with hyperthyroidism [5]. Meta-analyses of cohort studies have revealed an excess risk of fractures in people with subclinical hyperthyroidism [3, 4, 6], and even in populations with high-normal free thyroxine (FT4) and low-normal thyrotropin (thyroid-stimulating hormone, TSH), according to current reference ranges [7].

The association of even mild severities of hyperthyroidism with bone loss and increased fracture risk raises a question over the possibility of an adverse effect on the skeleton of either over treatment with LT4, or during receipt of the TSH-suppressive doses of LT4 administered following the surgical removal of thyroid tumours. This chapter reviews clinical studies of bone health in people receiving treatment with LT4 in these settings.

2 Bone Health in Patients Receiving Treatment with Levothyroxine

2.1 Patients with Congenital Hypothyroidism

Early and continuous treatment with LT4 has been shown to promote normal growth [8, 9] and BMD or other indices of bone health [10–12] in children with congenital hypothyroidism, relative to their euthyroid peers (Fig. 1), and normal BMD in adults [13]. Maintenance of a healthy weight and calcium intake appears to be an important determinant of bone health in these children, as in other populations [11].

2.2 Adult Patients with Hypothyroidism

2.2.1 Subclinical Hypothyroidism

Administration of LT4 to women with subclinical hypothyroidism increased the rate of bone turnover although whether this effect of LT4 *per se*, or a reversal of a previous hypothyroid-induced reduction in bone turnover was unclear [14]. A meta-analysis of studies in populations with subclinical hypothyroidism found no clinically significant reduction in bone loss during LT4 treatment in pre-menopausal women (2.7% after 8.5 years of treatment), but there was more significant bone loss in post-menopausal women (9.0% after 9.9 years of treatment) [15]. In contrast, a randomised, controlled trial found no effect of 14 months of LT4

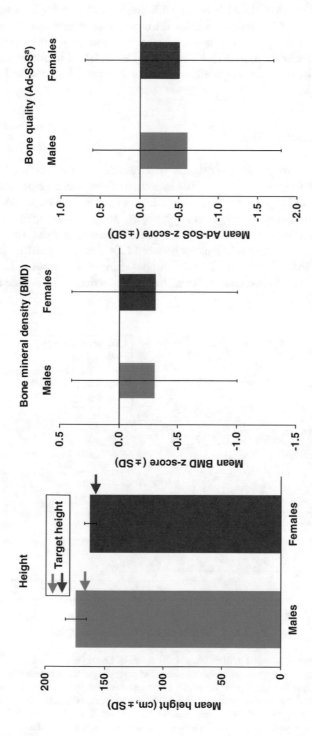

Fig. 1 Mean height and z-scores for bone mineral density and bone quality in adolescent/early adult subjects with congenital hypothyroidism treated early and continuously from birth with levothyroxine. [a]Ad-Sos is "amplitude-dependent speed of sound" in bone, a measure of bone quality. Measurements were made in 12 males and 25 females (mean age 18 ± 1 year). (Drawn from data presented in Ref. [9])

vs. no treatment on BMD in 17 women with subclinical hypothyroidism [16]. Observational data over 3 years showed that the bone-preserving effect of hormone replacement therapy for post-menopausal women was blunted during administration of LT4 for subclinical hypothyroidism [17]. Finally, BMD in adolescent girls treated with LT4 for subclinical hypothyroidism for 2–5 years had similar BMD to a control group [18].

2.2.2 Overt Hypothyroidism

LT4 dosage >150 mg/day, vs. lower doses, was associated with increased risk of fractures in women aged ≥65 years with hypothyroidism and a prior history of osteoporosis (Fig. 2) [19]. There was no significant effect in women without prior osteoporosis in this study. Another cross-sectional, observational study in post-menopausal women found reduced BMD associated with a longer duration of LT4 treatment, with no significant relationship between LT4 dosage and BMD in these women [20]. Another observational study in post-menopausal women found no association between LT4 treatment and bone loss, irrespective of the degree of suppression of TSH [21].

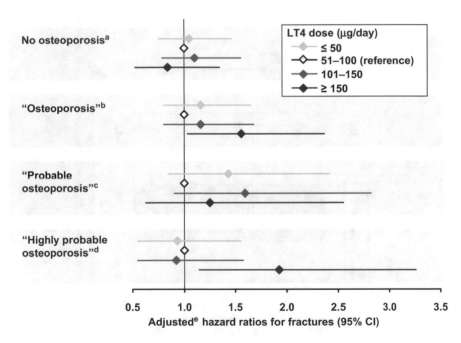

Fig. 2 Risk of fractures associated with different daily doses of levothyroxine in a large database population stratified by osteoporosis status at baseline. [a]No prior diagnosis of osteoporosis and no prescriptions for bisphosphonates; [b]prior diagnosis of osteoporosis regardless of treatment; [c]prior diagnosis of osteoporosis without prescription of bisphosphonate or raloxifene; [d]prior diagnosis of osteoporosis with prescription of bisphosphonate or raloxifene; [e]for age, comorbidities, co-medications, Charlson comorbidity score, health service usage. (Drawn from data presented in Ref. [19])

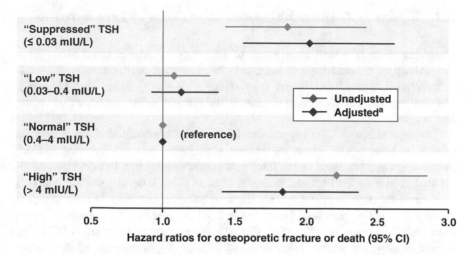

Fig. 3 Risk of a composite outcome of osteoporotic fractures or death, according to the prevailing level of thyrotropin (TSH), in a population-based database study of individuals receiving treatment with levothyroxine from the UK. ᵃAdjusted for age, gender, history of hyperthyroidism, history of osteoporotic fracture, presence or absence of diabetes. (Drawn from data presented in Ref. [22])

Large database studies have also evaluated the effect of LT4 treatment on bone in general populations of patients with hypothyroidism. In one study, patients receiving LT4 therapy were at increased risk of fractures if they had either a high TSH level (>4 mIU/L) or a suppressed TSH level (≤0.03 mIU/L), compared with patients with TSH within the reference range (Fig. 3) [22]. Patients with TSH 0.4–4.0 mIU/L were not at increased risk of fractures in this study. Another large database study of 162,369 people with hypothyroidism, of whom 97% received LT4 during follow-up, found increased fracture risk among those with TSH >10 mIU/L, compared with those well controlled to within the euthyroid range (HR 1.15 (95%CI 1.01–1.31, $p = 0.03$) [23]. These studies demonstrated the importance of optimisation of LT4 treatment, rather than LT4 treatment *per se*, for maintaining bone health.

A case-control study from Denmark, where all 124,655 patients with a fracture served as cases and 373,962 randomly selected age- and gender-matched people without fractures served as controls, found no association between LT4 treatment and risk of fracture [24]. An analysis of 23,183 LT4 users from the UK General Practice Research Database (i.e. managed in the primary care setting) also found no significant association between LT4 use and fracture risk overall although there was an apparent increased risk in males [25]. Other observational data also did not identify a significant effect of LT4 treatment on bone health [26].

The recent SORTED 1 trial found no difference in effects on bone health measured using circulating levels of C-terminal telopeptide (CTx) levels in very elderly patients (≥80 years) with hypothyroidism randomised to control of TSH in the standard reference range (0.4–4.0 mIU/L), or to a higher target range (4.1–8.0 mIU/L) [27]; see chapter, "Levothyroxine in the Older Patient" for a fuller account of this trial. CTx correlates inversely with TSH, including during treatment with LT4, and may provide a useful marker for following effects of LT4 on bone metabolism [28].

2.3   Effects of Thyrotropin-Suppressive Doses of Levothyroxine

Long-term treatment with high doses of LT4 may be administered to suppress the activity of residual thyroid tumour cells after total thyroidectomy for well-differentiated thyroid carcinoma (see chapter, "Levothyroxine and Cancer"). This setting has been likened to a state of "subclinical hyperthyroidism" by some authors [29].

The application of TSH-suppressive doses of LT4 has raised concern over its effects on bone health, given the known association between hyperthyroidism, osteoporosis and increased risk of fractures, as described above. Indeed, many clinical studies have applied various measures of bone mineral density or other markers of skeletal function to post-surgical, athyroid patients receiving TSH-suppressive therapy. Conflicting results of the effects of TSH suppression were reported in pre-menopausal women (adverse effect [30–41], or no clear adverse effect [42–47]), or post-menopausal women (adverse effect [40, 48, 49] or no clear adverse effect [31, 45, 47, 50–53]). Clear adverse safety signals for osteoporosis during TSH suppression did not emerge from several studies in populations that included female populations of mixed pre-/post-menopausal status [54–60], men [31, 45, 61–63] or a mixture of either gender [37, 64–67] (one small study in a mixed population demonstrated increased bone loss with TSH suppression in patients with thyroid cancer [68]). Trabecular bone score may be a more sensitive measure than bone mineral density of the effects of treatment with LT4 on bone structure this parameter has been used in patients who have [31, 32], or have not [69], received thyroidectomy and TSH suppression for thyroid cancer, although changes in this measure did not correlate with changes in BMD in LT4-treated patients in another study [70]. An absence of marked effects on bone health was also observed in studies in which pre-menopausal women [71–74], post-menopausal women [71, 74, 75] or mixed populations [76, 77] received less intensive TSH-suppressive therapy for benign thyroid nodules, or for goitre.

Several studies evaluated fracture risk. One study found that the 10-year fracture risk (assessed using FRAX, an online risk assessment tool) in women (mean age 52 years) did not correlate significantly with LT4 dose, the duration of LT4 therapy or FT4 [42]. Others found no marked increase in the risk of fractures associated with TSH-suppressive therapy [65, 78, 79]. One study found associations between the intensity of TSH suppression and fracture risk: the incidence of vertebral fractures was 45% for patients with TSH <0.5 mIU/L, compared with 24% for TSH 0.5–1.0 mIU/L and 4% for TSH >1.0 mIU/L [80]. Similarly, the risk of osteoporosis was increased in patients receiving a cumulative LT4 dose over time of >395 mg, but not in patients receiving a lower dose, among 9398 patients with new-onset thyroid cancer followed for an average of 6.6 years [81].

Determinants of bone health in patients receiving TSH-suppressive therapy appear to be complex and multifactorial. A family history of osteoporosis and oestrogen deficiency have been identified as risk factors for adverse effects on bone in this population [57, 58, 82]. TSH-suppressive therapy itself was shown not to affect levels of sex hormone-binding globulin [83]. More data on the relationship of TSH-suppressive therapy and bone health are required, relating to older subjects, and men, in particular, however [84].

3 Clinical Perspectives

Clinical data on the effects of LT4 administration on bone are conflicting. The many studies reviewed above differed importantly in design, their populations, their durations and the indices of bone health measured, especially with regard to important clinical outcomes, such as fractures. In general, the use of LT4 to maintain euthyroid levels of thyroid hormones in patients with hypothyroidism, or even the use of TSH-suppressive therapy following removal of thyroid tumours, does not appear to carry a substantial risk of osteoporosis or fractures. Nevertheless, the associations between LT4 administration and loss of bone mineralisation of increased fracture risk in some studies suggests the use of a cautious approach to avoid over treatment, especially in patients with or at risk of developing osteoporosis, such as postmenopausal women, or the elderly.

References

1. Bassett JH, Williams GR. Role of thyroid hormones in skeletal development and bone maintenance. Endocr Rev. 2016;37:135–87.
2. Williams GR, Bassett JHD. Thyroid diseases and bone health. J Endocrinol Investig. 2018;41:99–109.
3. Yang R, Du C, Xu J, Yao L, Zhang S, Wu Y. The relationship between subclinical thyroid dysfunction and the risk of fracture or low bone mineral density: a systematic review and meta-analysis of cohort studies. J Bone Miner Metab. 2018;36:209–20.
4. Yan Z, Huang H, Li J, Wang J. Relationship between subclinical thyroid dysfunction and the risk of fracture: a meta-analysis of prospective cohort studies. Osteoporos Int. 2016;27:115–25.
5. Vestergaard P, Mosekilde L. Hyperthyroidism, bone mineral, and fracture risk—a meta-analysis. Thyroid. 2003;13:585–93.
6. Blum MR, Bauer DC, Collet TH, et al. Subclinical thyroid dysfunction and fracture risk: a meta-analysis. JAMA. 2015;313:2055–65.
7. Aubert CE, Floriani C, Bauer DC, et al. Thyroid function tests in the reference range and fracture: individual participant analysis of prospective cohorts. J Clin Endocrinol Metab. 2017;102:2719–28.
8. Uyttendaele M, Lambert S, Tenoutasse S, et al. Congenital hypothyroidism: long-term experience with early and high levothyroxine dosage. Horm Res Paediatr. 2016;85:188–97.
9. Salerno M, Lettiero T, Esposito-del Puente A, et al. Effect of long-term L-thyroxine treatment on bone mineral density in young adults with congenital hypothyroidism. Eur J Endocrinol. 2004;151:689–94.
10. Pitukcheewanont P, Safani D, Gilsanz V, Klein M, Chongpison Y, Costin G. Quantitative computed tomography measurements of bone mineral density in prepubertal children with congenital hypothyroidism treated with L-thyroxine. J Pediatr Endocrinol Metab. 2004;17:889–93.

11. Leger J, Ruiz JC, Guibourdenche J, Kindermans C, Garabedian M, Czernichow P. Bone mineral density and metabolism in children with congenital hypothyroidism after prolonged L-thyroxine therapy. Acta Paediatr. 1997;86:704–10.
12. Kooh SW, Brnjac L, Ehrlich RM, Qureshi R, Krishnan S. Bone mass in children with congenital hypothyroidism treated with thyroxine since birth. J Pediatr Endocrinol Metab. 1996;9:59–62.
13. Kempers MJ, Vulsma T, Wiedijk BM, de Vijlder JJ, van Eck-Smit BL, Verberne HJ. The effect of life-long thyroxine treatment and physical activity on bone mineral density in young adult women with congenital hypothyroidism. Pediatr Endocrinol Metab. 2006;19:1405–12.
14. Meier C, Beat M, Guglielmetti M, Christ-Crain M, Staub JJ, Kraenzlin M. Restoration of euthyroidism accelerates bone turnover in patients with subclinical hypothyroidism: a randomized controlled trial. Osteoporos Int. 2004;15:209–16.
15. Faber J, Galløe AM. Changes in bone mass during prolonged subclinical hyperthyroidism due to L-thyroxine treatment: a meta-analysis. Eur J Endocrinol. 1994;130:350–6.
16. Ross DS. Bone density is not reduced during the short-term administration of levothyroxine to postmenopausal women with subclinical hypothyroidism: a randomized, prospective study. Am J Med. 1993;95:385–8.
17. Pines A, Dotan I, Tabori U, et al. L-thyroxine prevents the bone-conserving effect of HRT in postmenopausal women with subclinical hypothyroidism. Gynecol Endocrinol. 1999;13:196–201.
18. Saggese G, Bertelloni S, Baroncelli GI, Costa S, Ceccarelli C. Bone mineral density in adolescent females treated with L-thyroxine: a longitudinal study. Eur J Pediatr. 1996;155:452–7.
19. Ko YJ, Kim JY, Lee J, et al. Levothyroxine dose and fracture risk according to the osteoporosis status in elderly women. J Prev Med Public Health. 2014;47:36–46.
20. Affinito P, Sorrentino C, Farace MJ, et al. Effects of thyroxine therapy on bone metabolism in postmenopausal women with hypothyroidism. Acta Obstet Gynecol Scand. 1996;75:843–8.
21. Grant DJ, McMurdo ME, Mole PA, Paterson CR, Davies RR. Suppressed TSH levels secondary to thyroxine replacement therapy are not associated with osteoporosis. Clin Endocrinol (Oxf). 1993;39:529–33.
22. Flynn RW, Bonellie SR, Jung RT, MacDonald TM, Morris AD, Leese GP. Serum thyroid-stimulating hormone concentration and morbidity from cardiovascular disease and fractures in patients on long-term thyroxine therapy. J Clin Endocrinol Metab. 2010;95:186–93.
23. Thayakaran R, Adderley NJ, Sainsbury C, et al. Thyroid replacement therapy, thyroid stimulating hormone concentrations, and long term health outcomes in patients with hypothyroidism: longitudinal study. BMJ. 2019;366:l4892.
24. Vestergaard P, Rejnmark L, Mosekilde L. Influence of hyper- and hypothyroidism, and the effects of treatment with antithyroid drugs and levothyroxine on fracture risk. Calcif Tissue Int. 2005;77:139–44.
25. Sheppard MC, Holder R, Franklyn JA. Levothyroxine treatment and occurrence of fracture of the hip. Arch Intern Med. 2002;162:338–43.
26. Fowler PB, McIvor J, Sykes L, Macrae KD. The effect of long-term thyroxine on bone mineral density and serum cholesterol. J R Coll Physicians Lond. 1996;30:527–32.
27. Razvi S, Ryan V, Ingoe L, Pearce SH, Wilkes S. Age-related serum thyroid-stimulating hormone reference range in older patients treated with levothyroxine: a randomized controlled feasibility trial (SORTED 1). Eur Thyroid J. 2020;9:40–8.
28. Christy AL, D'Souza V, Babu RP, et al. Utility of C-terminal telopeptide in evaluating levothyroxine replacement therapy-induced bone loss. Biomark Insights. 2014;9:1–6.
29. Biondi B, Cooper DS. Benefits of thyrotropin suppression versus the risks of adverse effects in differentiated thyroid cancer. Thyroid. 2010;20:135–46.
30. Bin-Hong D, Fu-Man D, Yu L, Xu-Ping W, Bing-Feng B. Effects of levothyroxine therapy on bone mineral density and bone turnover markers in premenopausal women with thyroid cancer after thyroidectomy. Endokrynol Pol. 2020;71:15–20.
31. Moon JH, Kim KM, Oh TJ, et al. The effect of TSH suppression on vertebral trabecular bone scores in patients with differentiated thyroid carcinoma. J Clin Endocrinol Metab. 2017;102:78–85.

32. De Mingo Dominguez ML, Guadalix Iglesias S, Martin-Arriscado Arroba C, et al. Low trabecular bone score in postmenopausal women with differentiated thyroid carcinoma after long-term TSH suppressive therapy. Endocrine. 2018;62:166–73.
33. Kim MK, Yun KJ, Kim MH, et al. The effects of thyrotropin-suppressing therapy on bone metabolism in patients with well-differentiated thyroid carcinoma. Bone. 2015;71:101–5.
34. Schneider R, Schneider M, Reiners C, Schneider P. Effects of levothyroxine on bone mineral density, muscle force, and bone turnover markers: a cohort study. J Clin Endocrinol Metab. 2012;97:3926–34.
35. Sugitani I, Fujimoto Y. Effect of postoperative thyrotropin suppressive therapy on bone mineral density in patients with papillary thyroid carcinoma: a prospective controlled study. Surgery. 2011;150:1250–7.
36. Mazokopakis EE, Starakis IK, Papadomanolaki MG, Batistakis AG, Papadakis JA. Changes of bone mineral density in pre-menopausal women with differentiated thyroid cancer receiving L-thyroxine suppressive therapy. Curr Med Res Opin. 2006;22:1369–73.
37. Karner I, Hrgović Z, Sijanović S, et al. Bone mineral density changes and bone turnover in thyroid carcinoma patients treated with supraphysiologic doses of thyroxine. Eur J Med Res. 2005;10:480–8.
38. Guang-Da X, Hui-Ling S, Zhi-Song C, Lin-Shuang Z. Alteration of plasma concentrations of OPG before and after levothyroxine replacement therapy in hypothyroid patients. J Endocrinol Investig. 2005;28:965–72.
39. Marcocci C, Golia F, Bruno-Bossio G, Vignali E, Pinchera A. Carefully monitored levothyroxine suppressive therapy is not associated with bone loss in premenopausal women. J Clin Endocrinol Metab. 1994;78:818–23.
40. Jódar E, Begoña López M, García L, Rigopoulou D, Martínez G, Hawkins F. Bone changes in pre- and postmenopausal women with thyroid cancer on levothyroxine therapy: evolution of axial and appendicular bone mass. Osteoporos Int. 1998;8:311–6.
41. Pioli G, Pedrazzoni M, Palummeri E, et al. Longitudinal study of bone loss after thyroidectomy and suppressive thyroxine therapy in premenopausal women. Acta Endocrinol (Copenh). 1992;126:238–42.
42. Vera L, Gay S, Campomenosi C, et al. Ten-year estimated risk of bone fracture in women with differentiated thyroid cancer under TSH-suppressive levothyroxine therapy. Endokrynol Pol. 2016;67:350 8.
43. Kim CW, Hong S, Oh SH, et al. Change of bone mineral density and biochemical markers of bone turnover in patients on suppressive levothyroxine therapy for differentiated thyroid carcinoma. J Bone Metab. 2015;22:135–41.
44. Mendonça Monteiro de Barros G, Madeira M, Vieira Neto L, et al. Bone mineral density and bone microarchitecture after long-term suppressive levothyroxine treatment of differentiated thyroid carcinoma in young adult patients. J Bone Miner Metab. 2016;34:417–21.
45. Eftekhari M, Asadollahi A, Beiki D, et al. The long term effect of levothyroxine on bone mineral density in patients with well differentiated thyroid carcinoma after treatment. Hell J Nucl Med. 2008;11:160–3.
46. Sajjinanont T, Rajchadara S, Sriassawaamorn N, Panichkul S. The comparative study of bone mineral density between premenopausal women receiving long term suppressive doses of levothyroxine for well-differentiated thyroid cancer with healthy premenopausal women. J Med Assoc Thail. 2005;88(Suppl 3):S71–6.
47. Görres G, Kaim A, Otte A, Götze M, Müller-Brand J. Bone mineral density in patients receiving suppressive doses of thyroxine for differentiated thyroid carcinoma. Eur J Nucl Med. 1996;23:690–2.
48. Giannini S, Nobile M, Sartori L, et al. Bone density and mineral metabolism in thyroidectomized patients treated with long-term L-thyroxine. Clin Sci (Lond). 1994;87:593–7.
49. Kung AW, Lorentz T, Tam SC. Thyroxine suppressive therapy decreases bone mineral density in post-menopausal women. Clin Endocrinol (Oxf). 1993;39:535–40.
50. Zhang P, Xi H, Yan R. Effects of thyrotropin suppression on lumbar bone mineral density in postmenopausal women with differentiated thyroid carcinoma. Onco Targets Ther. 2018;11:6687–92.

51. de Melo TG, da Assumpção LV, Santos Ade O, Zantut-Wittmann DE. Low BMI and low TSH value as risk factors related to lower bone mineral density in postmenospausal women under levothyroxine therapy for differentiated thyroid carcinoma. Thyroid Res. 2015;8:7.
52. Fujiyama K, Maki H, Kinoshita S, Yoshida T. Suppressive doses of thyroxine do not accelerate age-related bone loss in late postmenopausal women. Thyroid. 1995;5:13–7.
53. Hawkins F, Rigopoulou D, Papapietro K, Lopez MB. Spinal bone mass after long-term treatment with L-thyroxine in postmenopausal women with thyroid cancer and chronic lymphocytic thyroiditis. Calcif Tissue Int. 1994;54:16–9.
54. Lee MY, Park JH, Bae KS, et al. Bone mineral density and bone turnover markers in patients on long-term suppressive levothyroxine therapy for differentiated thyroid cancer. Ann Surg Treat Res. 2014;86:55–60.
55. Reverter JL, Holgado S, Alonso N, Salinas I, Granada ML, Sanmartí A. Lack of deleterious effect on bone mineral density of long-term thyroxine suppressive therapy for differentiated thyroid carcinoma. Endocr Relat Cancer. 2005;12:973–81.
56. Chen CH, Wang PH, Chiu LH, Chang WH. Bone mineral density in women receiving thyroxine suppressive therapy for differentiated thyroid carcinoma. Formos Med Assoc. 2004;103:442–7.
57. Mikosch P, Jauk B, Gallowitsch HJ, Pipam W, Kresnik E, Lind P. Suppressive levothyroxine therapy has no significant influence on bone degradation in women with thyroid carcinoma: a comparison with other disorders affecting bone metabolism. Thyroid. 2001;11:257–63.
58. Mikosch P, Obermayer-Pietsch B, Jost R, et al. Bone metabolism in patients with differentiated thyroid carcinoma receiving suppressive levothyroxine treatment. Thyroid. 2003;13:347–56.
59. Müller CG, Bayley TA, Harrison JE, Tsang R. Possible limited bone loss with suppressive thyroxine therapy is unlikely to have clinical relevance. Thyroid. 1995;5:81–7.
60. Florkowski CM, Brownlie BE, Elliot JR, Ayling EM, Turner JG. Bone mineral density in patients receiving suppressive doses of thyroxine for thyroid carcinoma. N Z Med J. 1993;106:443–4.
61. Reverter JL, Colomé E, Holgado S, et al. Bone mineral density and bone fracture in male patients receiving long-term suppressive levothyroxine treatment for differentiated thyroid carcinoma. Endocrine. 2010;37:467–72.
62. Jódar E, Martínez-Díaz-Guerra G, Azriel S, Hawkins F. Bone mineral density in male patients with L-thyroxine suppressive therapy and Graves disease. Calcif Tissue Int. 2001;69:84–7.
63. Marcocci C, Golia F, Vignali E, Pinchera A. Skeletal integrity in men chronically treated with suppressive doses of L-thyroxine. J Bone Miner Res. 1997;12:72–7.
64. Kachui A, Tabatabaizadeh SM, Iraj B, Rezvanian H, Feizi A. Evaluation of bone density, serum total and ionized calcium, alkaline phosphatase and 25-hydroxy vitamin D in papillary thyroid carcinoma, and their relationship with TSH suppression by levothyroxine. Adv Biomed Res. 2017;6:94.
65. Heijckmann AC, Huijberts MS, Geusens P, de Vries J, Menheere PP, Wolffenbuttel BH. Hip bone mineral density, bone turnover and risk of fracture in patients on long-term suppressive L-thyroxine therapy for differentiated thyroid carcinoma. Eur J Endocrinol. 2005;153:23–9.
66. Rosen HN, Moses AC, Garber J, et al. Randomized trial of pamidronate in patients with thyroid cancer: bone density is not reduced by suppressive doses of thyroxine, but is increased by cyclic intravenous pamidronate. J Clin Endocrinol Metab. 1998;83:2324–30.
67. Franklyn JA, Betteridge J, Daykin J, et al. Long-term thyroxine treatment and bone mineral density. Lancet. 1992;340:9–13.
68. MT MD, Perloff JJ, Kidd GS. A longitudinal assessment of bone loss in women with levothyroxine-suppressed benign thyroid disease and thyroid cancer. Calcif Tissue Int. 1995;56:521–5.
69. Hwangbo Y, Kim JH, Kim SW, et al. High-normal free thyroxine levels are associated with low trabecular bone scores in euthyroid postmenopausal women. Osteoporos Int. 2016;27:457–62.
70. Kim K, Kim IJ, Pak K, et al. Evaluation of bone mineral density using dxa and cqct in postmenopausal patients under thyrotropin suppressive therapy. J Clin Endocrinol Metab. 2018;103:4232–40.

71. Appetecchia M. Effects on bone mineral density by treatment of benign nodular goiter with mildly suppressive doses of L-thyroxine in a cohort women study. Horm Res. 2005;64:293–8.
72. Larijani B, Gharibdoost F, Pajouhi M, et al. Effects of levothyroxine suppressive therapy on bone mineral density in premenopausal women. J Clin Pharm Ther. 2004;29:1–5.
73. Nuzzo V, Lupoli G, Esposito Del Puente A, et al. Bone mineral density in premenopausal women receiving levothyroxine suppressive therapy. Gynecol Endocrinol. 1998;12:333–7.
74. De Rosa G, Testa A, Maussier ML, Callà C, Astazi P, Albanese C. A slightly suppressive dose of L-thyroxine does not affect bone turnover and bone mineral density in pre- and postmeno-pausal women with nontoxic goitre. Horm Metab Res. 1995;27:503–7.
75. Chen CY, Chen ST, Huang BY, Hwang JS, Lin JD, Liu FH. The effect of suppressive thyroxine therapy in nodular goiter in postmenopausal women and 2 year's bone mineral density change. Endocr J. 2018;65:1101–9.
76. Baldini M, Serafino S, Zanaboni L, Cappellini MD. Treatment of benign nodular goitre with mildly suppressive doses of L-thyroxine: effects on bone mineral density and on nodule size. J Intern Med. 2002;251:407–14.
77. Zelmanovitz F, Genro S, Gross JL. Suppressive therapy with levothyroxine for solitary thyroid nodules: a double-blind controlled clinical study and cumulative meta-analyses. J Clin Endocrinol Metab. 1998;83:3881–5.
78. Nguyen TT, Heath H 3rd, Bryant SC, O'Fallon WM, Melton LJ 3rd. Fractures after thyroidectomy in men: a population-based cohort study. J Bone Miner Res. 1997;12:1092–9.
79. Melton LJ 3rd, Ardila E, Crowson CS, O'Fallon WM, Khosla S. Fractures following thyroidectomy in women: a population-based cohort study. Bone. 2000;27:695–700.
80. Mazziotti G, Formenti AM, Frara S, et al. High prevalence of radiological vertebral fractures in women on thyroid-stimulating hormone-suppressive therapy for thyroid carcinoma. J Clin Endocrinol Metab. 2018;103:956–64.
81. Lin SY, Lin CL, Chen HT, Kao CH. Risk of osteoporosis in thyroid cancer patients using levothyroxine: a population-based study. Curr Med Res Opin. 2018;34:805–12.
82. Soydal Ç, Özkan E, Nak D, Elhan AH, Küçük NÖ, Kır MK. Risk factors for predicting osteoporosis in patients who receive thyrotropin suppressive levothyroxine treatment for differentiated thyroid carcinoma. Mol Imaging Radionucl Ther. 2019;28:69–75.
83. Lecomte P, Lecureuil N, Osorio-Salazar C, Lecureuil M, Valat C. Effects of suppressive doses of levothyroxine treatment on sex-hormone-binding globulin and bone metabolism. Thyroid. 1995;5:19–23.
84. Papaleontiou M, Hawley ST, Haymart MR. Effect of thyrotropin suppression therapy on bone in thyroid cancer patients. Oncologist. 2016;21:165–71.

Levothyroxine and Cancer

Tomasz Bednarczuk

Treatment with LT4 is used to suppress thyrotropin levels after the management of differentiated thyroid cancers after surgery, with doses and targets for thyrotropin (thyroid-stimulating hormone, TSH) determined by the risk of cancer recurrence determined in the individual patient. Moreover, the role of thyroid hormones and their receptors in the initiation—and, potentially, cure—of a range of cancer types is an active area of research.

1 Introduction

1.1 Overview of the Management of Differentiated Thyroid Cancer

In general, the treatment of differentiated thyroid cancers (DTC) consists of surgery, post-operative/adjuvant radioactive iodine (RAI, ^{131}I) treatment and hormonal therapy with levothyroxine (LT4) [1, 2]. Surgery is the standard intervention for the management of DTC (although the management of microcancers of the thyroid remains a matter of debate) [1, 2]. Where the patient receives a total thyroidectomy, the resulting athyroid state induces a severe hypothyroidism that causes thyrotropin (TSH) to rise to high levels, typically at least 30 IU/mL after several weeks (compared with the usual upper limit of the normal reference range of about 4 mIU/L) [3].

For papillary or follicular thyroid tumours, the high TSH level stimulates any remaining unresectable thyroid tissue or metastatic tumour cells that retain some

T. Bednarczuk (✉)
Department of Internal Diseases and Endocrinology, Medical University of Warsaw, Warsaw, Poland
e-mail: tbednarczuk@wum.edu.pl

© The Author(s) 2021
G. J. Kahaly (ed.), *70 Years of Levothyroxine*,
https://doi.org/10.1007/978-3-030-63277-9_9

endocrine activity to take up iodine from the circulation [3]. Treatment with RAI is then administered periodically over a period of years and the RAI is taken up avidly by these cells resulting in their irradiation and ablation: in this way, the majority of these cancers can be eradicated successfully [1, 3]. Injections of recombinant human TSH may also be used to increase RAI uptake of residual thyroid cancer cells [3, 4].

Patients may require lifelong substitution of LT4 after thyroid surgery for DTC, depending on the amount of thyroid tissue removed [3, 5]. Moreover, high-risk patients may receive TSH-suppressive therapy with LT4. The decision on whether to aim for full suppression of TSH (TSH < 0.1 mIU/L), or partial TSH suppression (TSH 0.1–0.4 mIU/L) should be personalised [2, 3].

1.2 Scope of This Chapter

This chapter reviews the benefits and risks associated with LT4-suppressive therapy in patients who have undergone surgery and RAI for DTC. The diagnosis of thyroid cancer, tumour staging, allocation of patients to different modalities of surgery and their outcomes, and the application, effectiveness of and development of refractoriness to RAI *per se* are beyond its scope and will not be discussed further here (we refer the reader to current guidelines in these areas [1, 3, 5, 6]). In addition, the consequences of long-term suppressive LT4 administration for bone homeostasis and health in these patients are considered in chapter "Levothyroxine and Bone" of this book, and are also not discussed in detail here. Chapter "Levothyroxine and the Heart" of this book reviews the effects of TSH-suppressive doses of LT4 on the heart. Finally, medullary thyroid tumours arise from calcitonin-secreting parafollicular cells (C-cells) that do not secrete thyroxine: these patients are not treated with RAI and LT4 and their management is also not addressed here [7].

2 Application of Thyrotropin-Suppressive Doses of Levothyroxine After Surgery and Radioactive Iodine for Well-Differentiated Thyroid Tumours

2.1 Need for Suppression of Thyrotropin in Thyroid Cancer Survivors

TSH promotes the growth of thyroid tumours, and levels of this hormone are suppressed in the initial period following surgery for many DTC. A meta-analysis supports the effectiveness of this approach in improving long-term clinical outcomes post-thyroidectomy, compared with patients who did not receive TSH-suppressive therapy [8]. However, it has become clear in recent years that stringent suppression of TSH does not improve long-term clinical outcomes in patients with other than high-risk presentations of well-differentiated thyroid cancer [9–13]. Accordingly, patients with thyroid cancer assessed as being at lower risk of disease recurrence do not require complete suppression of TSH. This approach is designed to optimise the balance between suppression of disease recurrence (benefit) and the potential for adverse effects on bone [9].

For adults, the level of thyroglobulin has been found to be strongly predictive of the risk of recurrent disease (see Fig. 1a) [14], and thus different targets for TSH suppression are provided in guidelines for low-risk patients according to their post-surgery thyroglobulin levels [1, 3]. A recent meta-analysis has confirmed the diagnostic and prognostic power of thyroglobulin measurement during post-thyroidectomy TSH suppression using LT4, with negative predictive value for ruling out evidence of structural thyroid carcinoma in excess of 99% [15]. The relationship between thyroglobulin and post-surgical outcome is less well understood in children, for whom targets for TSH suppression are accordingly not stratified formally according to the thyroglobulin level [3].

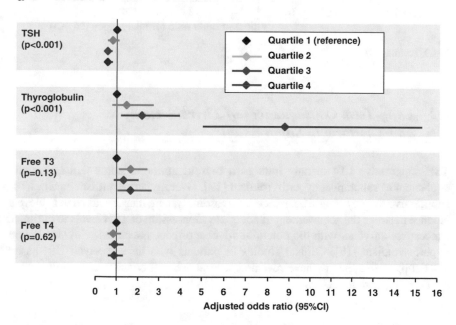

Fig. 1 Thyroid hormones homeostasis and the risk of thyroid cancer. (a) Case-control study from the EPIC cohort. A population of 357 individuals with differentiated thyroid cancer were matched with 2 (women) or 3 (men) cancer-free control subjects. Significance values shown are p for trend. Total thyroxine (T3) and total triiodothyronine (T3) did not significantly influence cancer risk and have been omitted for clarity. Adjusted for study site, age, gender, time/data of blood draw. (Drawn from data presented in Ref. [14]). (b) Risk factors for malignancy within the thyroid nodules in a multivariable logistic regression analysis that included variation of thyrotropin (TSH) levels within the normal range. Adjusted for gender, age, nodule size, preoperative TSH in patients not on levothyroxine. (Drawn from data presented in Ref. [26])

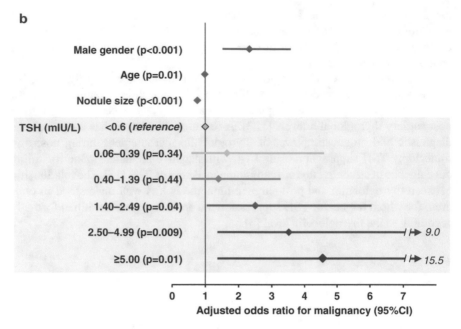

Fig. 1 (continued)

2.2 Long-Term Consequences of Thyroidectomy and Thyrotropin Suppression

TSH-suppressive LT4 therapy induces a thyroid hormone status that is broadly equivalent to subclinical hyperthyroidism [13]. Overt hyperthyroidism during LT4-suppressive therapy should be avoided. Accordingly, care must be taken to achieve a balance between the achievement of adequate suppression of TSH levels to optimise cancer-free survival, with the potential adverse effects associated with subclinical hyperthyroidism [16]. Clinical studies in patients who have received LT4-based TSH-suppressive therapy have revealed several areas of concern or benefit, which are described briefly below.

2.2.1 Bone

Untreated longstanding hyperthyroidism is associated with loss of bone mineralisation, osteoporosis and increased risk of fractures. Studies in TSH-suppressed populations have been conflicting, but some studies have demonstrated increased osteoporosis and fracture risk associated with LT4 treatment (reviewed in chapter "Levothyroxine and Bone" of this book).

2.2.2 The Cardiovascular System

A retrospective study from the Korean National Health Insurance database, which covers 97% of people in that country, evaluated the risk of coronary heart disease (CHD) and ischemic stroke over a follow-up period of 4.3 years in 182,419 patients following thyroidectomy for differentiated thyroid cancer [17]. Higher hazard ratios for CHD and stroke were found for the thyroidectomised population, relative to propensity score-matched controls. The signal for adverse cardiovascular outcomes became stronger at doses of LT4 that were higher than 115–144 μg/day. Although atrial fibrillation was more common in patients receiving higher doses of LT4, this was associated with only 4% of strokes. As expected, cardiovascular risk factors increased the risk of CHD or stroke. Another chart review in thyroid cancer survivors found no association between up to 9 years of over-suppression of TSH with LT4 (according to guideline recommendations based on risk of thyroid cancer recurrence) and adverse cardiovascular outcomes, but this study only contained 14 subjects [18]. Chapter "Levothyroxine and the Heart" of this book reviews the effects of LT4 on the heart.

2.2.3 Patient-Reported Outcomes

Fatigue is often reported as a long-term complication of thyroidectomy and subsequent TSH suppression [19]. One study showed that the persistence of residual symptoms reminiscent of hypothyroidism on TSH-suppressive therapy were correlated with a low level of FT3 [20]. Altering the dose of TSH, or switching to a combination of LT4 and T3 administration did not induce a clear improvement of fatigue, however [21, 22]. Current guidelines for the management of hypothyroidism recommend that LT4 remains the first-line treatment. Exercise appears to be an effective way of combating fatigue and improving the quality of life in this setting [21, 23]. A similar benefit was observed in LT4-treated breast cancer patients undergoing chemotherapy [24]. More clinical studies of this relatively common, and potentially disabling, complication of thyroid cancer management are needed [21].

3 Thyroid Hormones and Cancer Risk

Variations in thyroid hormones have been associated with changes in the risk of a wide range of cancer types [25]. Examples of effects of thyroid hormones on the risk of various tumour types in epidemiological studies are shown below. However, the results are often conflicting and have to be judged cautiously since association does not prove causation.

Thyroid: Observational data have associated an increased circulating level of TSH with an increased risk of developing differentiated thyroid cancer [26, 27] and/or a more advanced stage of this tumour at presentation [26]. Other studies found that low TSH increased the risk of thyroid cancer [14], that high TSH in men, but low TSH in women, was associated with thyroid cancer [28], or that the influence of abnormal TSH on cancer risk was amplified in non-diabetic subjects with higher levels of fasting serum glucose [29]. Fig. 1 shows the risk of cancer associated with thyroid nodules at different levels of TSH and other markers of thyroid homeostasis from two of these observational studies. Higher TSH levels were associated with a lower risk of incident differentiated thyroid cancer in one study (Fig. 1a) [14], while increases in TSH levels within the normal reference range increased thyroid cancer risk in the other study, in patients with thyroid nodules (Fig. 1b) [26].

Breast: Hyperthyroidism (high TT4 or FT4 and/or low TSH) has been associated with increased risk of breast cancer in some observational studies [30–32]. This association was shown to extend into the euthyroid range [33], and to be present pre- and post-menopause [34]. There was no effect of variation of TSH in other studies [31, 35], and the impact of anti-thyroid antibodies on breast cancer risk was variable [30–32]. A meta-analysis of 8 cross-sectional studies found a positive association between elevated T4, T3, anti-thyroid peroxidise antibodies and anti-thyroglobulin antibodies and the prevalence of breast cancer [36]. Likewise, autoimmune thyroiditis has been found to be more common in women with vs. without breast cancer [37].

A population-based case-control study from Taiwan (65,491 breast cancers, 261,964 controls) found that LT4 administration vs. no LT4 use was associated with a modestly higher risk of breast cancer, with a greater effect in older ($\geq$65 years) patients (odds ratio [OR] 1.45 [95%CI 1.23–1.71], $p < 0.01$) compared with younger patients (OR 1.19 [95%CI 1.09–1.29], $p < 0.01$) [38]. However, the ORs were similar for patients who received LT4 for $\leq$1 year (1.22) and >1 year (1.26), and further study is required to confirm this association.

Prostate: Low TSH/high T4 increased the risk of prostate cancer in a population-based observational study [30]. Conversely, and consistent with this study, high TSH was protective against prostate cancer in the population of a clinical trial conducted to answer a clinical question that was unrelated to thyroid function [39].

Gastrointestinal: A population-based study found no effect of TSH or FT4 levels on colorectal cancer risk [30]. However, high FT4, but not a diagnosis of hypothyroidism or hyperthyroidism, predicted shorter survival in a cohort of 258 patients with advanced gastro-oesophageal cancer [40]. Low FT3 was associated with prolonged survival in this study, which is difficult to reconcile with the adverse effect of high FT4 [40].

A large population-based case-control study from a UK general practice database (The Health Improvement Network, 20,990 colorectal cancer cases and 82,054 controls) found that both hyperthyroidism and untreated hypothyroidism predicted an increased risk of having colorectal cancer [41]. Long-term treatment with LT4 was associated with a reduced risk of colorectal cancer, with a lower risk for a longer treatment duration [41].

Liver: Higher TSH was associated with larger tumours in a cohort of 838 patients with advanced hepatocellular carcinoma, and higher FT4 ($\geq$16.6 ng/L) predicted poorer survival vs. lower levels of FT4 [42].

Pancreas: A retrospective study found that survival with pancreatic cancer did not vary according to hypothyroid or euthyroid status overall, but that hypothyroid patients taking LT4 demonstrated higher tumour stage, and more localised and distant tumour spread than euthyroid patients [43]. However, this study is difficult to interpret, as there were only 71 hypothyroid patients included, and there was no information presented on how many were taking LT4 [43].

Table 1 summarises briefly some potential mechanisms that have been demonstrated in clinical or experimental studies to explain an association between thyroid hormone status and tumorigenesis [44–67]. Thyroid hormones mediate their effects

Table 1 Potential mechanisms linking thyroid hormone actions to tumourigenesis or tumour suppression

Ref.	Potential mechanisms
	Promotion of invasion and metastasis
[44–47]	Promotion of proliferation of tumour cells or metastasis by altered intracellular downstream signalling pathways following interaction of T3 or T4 with a binding site on integrin αvβ3 in the extracellular matrix (breast, ovary)
[48, 49]	Promotion of metastasis and/or angiogenesis by enhanced epithelial-mesenchymal transition in tumour cells, also involving the integrin αvβ3–thyroid hormone axis
[50, 51]	Inhibition of apoptosis mediated via downstream signalling from thyroid hormone and other ligand binding sites on integrin αvβ3 (ovary)
[43]	Increased proliferation, migration, and invasion of pancreatic cancer cell lines in vitro after exposure to T3
[52]	Crosstalk between thyroid oestrogen receptors increased the growth of cancer cells, and this relationship was modulated by integrin αvβ3 (lung)
	Modulation of tumour cells
[53–55, 64]	Enhanced differentiation or renewal of cancer stem cells (colorectal, hepatocellular)
[65]	Release of inhibition of epigenetic regulation of gene expression reduced cancer cell growth (liver)
[56]	T3 may induce senescence in prostate cancer cells, which would oppose tumour growth
	Altered expression of thyroid hormone receptors α and β (TRα and TRβ)
[57, 58]	Expression of TRα drove tumour growth and worsened prognosis (breast)
[57, 59]	Higher expression of THRα2 receptor improved prognosis (breast)
[57, 59, 60, 63]	Expression of TRβ opposed tumour growth (breast)
[61, 62]	Suppression of the oncogenic RUNX2 transcription factor by increased expression of TRβ (breast, thyroid)
[63]	Cytoplasmic TRβ1 predicted improved survival, but nuclear TRβ1 predicted reduced survival (breast)
[64]	Activation of the T3/TRβ axis shifted hepatocellular tumour cells to a more benign, normal tissue-like phenotype
[60, 65, 66]	Reversal of epigenetic silencing of tumour suppressor genes via activation of thyroid receptors by T3 (thyroid, hepatocellular, kidney)
[67]	Reduced tumour growth by activation of the RhoB signalling pathway (thyroid)

on the cancer cell through several non-genomic pathways including activation of integrin avβ3 promoting metastasis and angiogenesis within tumours. Furthermore, cancer development and progression are affected by dysregulation of local bio-availability of thyroid hormones and thyroid hormone receptor changes [25, 45, 49, 68–70].

Tetraiodothyroacetic acid may oppose these actions [69]. The thyroid receptor, TRβ is downregulated in many tumours, and activation of this receptor has been proposed as a strategy for increasing the sensitivity of triple-negative breast cancer cells to chemotherapy [71].

Ovarian cancer is a highly metastatic tumour, and several thyroid hormone analogues exerted cytotoxic effects in ovarian cancer cell lines, probably by antagonising the effects of thyroid hormones on the integrin αvβ3 axis [72] A similar phenomenon has been observed in thyroid and lung cancer cells, among others [49, 51, 52, 69]. Tetraiodothyroacetic acid, a metabolite of T4, may reduce the resistance of cancer cells to radiotherapy [73]. Deiodinases modulate the local bioavailability of thyroid hormones, by controlling T4 conversion to T3 and other thyroid hormone derivatives and this expression of these enzymes differs in a range of tumour types, compared with non-neoplastic tissues [74, 75]. These observations provide promising avenues for future research on the development of novel anticancer agents.

4   Conclusions

Observational data have implicated variations in the levels of thyroid hormones with variations in the risk of a range of cancer types, including of the thyroid itself. This association extends to within the currently accepted "normal" range for thyroid hormones. In addition, the discovery of novel interactions between thyroid hormones and receptors both inside cells and in the extracellular space have opened up new avenues for anticancer research. Treatment with suppressive doses of LT4 is one of the key components of the management of differentiated thyroid cancers after surgery, where careful evaluation of the risk of cancer recurrence in the individual patient aids a balancing of the need to suppress TSH sufficiently with the need to avoid over treatment.

References

1. Filetti S, Durante C, Hartl D, et al. Thyroid cancer: ESMO clinical practice guidelines for diagnosis, treatment and follow-up. Ann Oncol. 2019;30:1856–83.
2. Jarząb B, Dedecjus M, Słowińska-Klencka D, et al. Guidelines of Polish National Societies diagnostics and treatment of thyroid carcinoma. 2018 update. Endokrynol Pol. 2018;69:34–74.
3. Haugen BR, Alexander EK, Bible KC, et al. 2015 American Thyroid Association management guidelines for adult patients with thyroid nodules and differentiated thyroid cancer: The

American Thyroid Association Guidelines Task Force on Thyroid Nodules and Differentiated Thyroid Cancer. Thyroid. 2016;26:1–133.

4. Giovanella L, Duntas LH. Management of endocrine disease: the role of rhTSH in the management of differentiated thyroid cancer: pros and cons. Eur J Endocrinol. 2019;181:R133–45.

5. Francis GL, Waguespack SG, Bauer AJ, et al. Management guidelines for children with thyroid nodules and differentiated thyroid cancer. Thyroid. 2015;25:716–59.

6. Fugazzola L, Elisei R, Fuhrer D, et al. 2019 European Thyroid Association guidelines for the treatment and follow-up of advanced radioiodine-refractory thyroid cancer. Eur Thyroid J. 2019;8:227–45.

7. Wells SA Jr, Asa SL, Dralle H, et al. Revised American Thyroid Association guidelines for the management of medullary thyroid carcinoma. Thyroid. 2015;25:567–610.

8. McGriff NJ, Csako G, Gourgiotis L, Lori CG, Pucino F, Sarlis NJ. Effects of thyroid hormone suppression therapy on adverse clinical outcomes in thyroid cancer. Ann Med. 2002;34:554–64.

9. Grani G, Ramundo V, Verrienti A, Sponziello M, Durante C. Thyroid hormone therapy in differentiated thyroid cancer. Endocrine. 2019;66:43–50.

10. Biondi B, Cooper DS. Thyroid hormone suppression therapy. Endocrinol Metab Clin N Am. 2019;48:227–37.

11. Lamartina L, Montesano T, Falcone R, et al. Is it worth suppressing TSH in low- and intermediate-risk papillary thyroid cancer patients before the first disease assessment? Endocr Pract. 2019;25:165–9.

12. Biondi B, Cooper DS. Benefits of thyrotropin suppression versus the risks of adverse effects in differentiated thyroid cancer. Thyroid. 2010;20:135–46.

13. Biondi B, Filetti S, Schlumberger M. Thyroid-hormone therapy and thyroid cancer: a reassessment. Nat Clin Pract Endocrinol Metab. 2005;1:32–40.

14. Rinaldi S, Plummer M, Biessy C, et al. Thyroid-stimulating hormone, thyroglobulin, and thyroid hormones and risk of differentiated thyroid carcinoma: the EPIC study. J Natl Cancer Inst. 2014;106:dju097.

15. Giovanella L, Castellana M, Trimboli P. Unstimulated high-sensitive thyroglobulin is a powerful prognostic predictor in patients with thyroid cancer. Clin Chem Lab Med. 2019;58:130–7.

16. Biondi B, Bartalena L, Cooper DS, Hegedüs L, Laurberg P, Kahaly GJ. The 2015 European Thyroid Association guidelines on diagnosis and treatment of endogenous subclinical hyperthyroidism. Eur Thyroid J. 2015;4:149–63.

17. Suh B, Shin DW, Park Y, et al. Increased cardiovascular risk in thyroid cancer patients taking levothyroxine: a nationwide cohort study in Korea. Eur J Endocrinol. 2019;180:11–20.

18. Hong KS, Son JW, Ryu OH, Choi MG, Hong JY, Lee SJ. Cardiac effects of thyrotropin oversuppression with levothyroxine in young women with differentiated thyroid cancer. Int J Endocrinol. 2016;2016:9846790.

19. Gamper EM, Wintner LM, Rodrigues M, et al. Persistent quality of life impairments in differentiated thyroid cancer patients: results from a monitoring programme. Eur J Nucl Med Mol Imaging. 2015;42:1179–88.

20. Larisch R, Midgley JEM, Dietrich JW, Hoermann R. Symptomatic relief is related to serum free triiodothyronine concentrations during follow-up in levothyroxine-treated patients with differentiated thyroid cancer. Exp Clin Endocrinol Diabetes. 2018;126:546–52.

21. To J, Goldberg AS, Jones J, et al. A systematic review of randomized controlled trials for management of persistent post-treatment fatigue in thyroid cancer survivors. Thyroid. 2015;25:198–210.

22. Massolt ET, van der Windt M, Korevaar TI, et al. Thyroid hormone and its metabolites in relation to quality of life in patients treated for differentiated thyroid cancer. Clin Endocrinol (Oxf). 2016;85:781–8.

23. Vigário Pdos S, Chachamovitz DS, Teixeira Pde F, Rocque Mde L, Santos ML, Vaisman M. Exercise is associated with better quality of life in patients on TSH-suppressive therapy with levothyroxine for differentiated thyroid carcinoma. Arq Bras Endocrinol Metabol. 2014;58:274–81.

24. Schmidt ME, Wiskemann J, Johnson T, Habermann N, Schneeweiss A, Steindorf K. L-Thyroxine intake as a potential risk factor for the development of fatigue in breast cancer patients undergoing chemotherapy. Support Care Cancer. 2018;26:2561–9.
25. Moeller LC, Führer D. Thyroid hormone, thyroid hormone receptors, and cancer: a clinical perspective. Endocr Relat Cancer. 2013;20:R19–29.
26. Haymart MR, Repplinger DJ, Leverson GE, et al. Higher serum thyroid stimulating hormone level in thyroid nodule patients is associated with greater risks of differentiated thyroid cancer and advanced tumor stage. J Clin Endocrinol Metab. 2008;93:809–14.
27. He LZ, Zeng TS, Pu L, Pan SX, Xia WF, Chen LL. Thyroid hormones, autoantibodies, ultrasonography, and clinical parameters for predicting thyroid cancer. Int J Endocrinol. 2016;2016:8215834.
28. Huang H, Rusiecki J, Zhao N, et al. Thyroid-stimulating hormone, thyroid hormones, and risk of papillary thyroid cancer: a nested case-control study. Cancer Epidemiol Biomark Prev. 2017;26:1209–18.
29. Hu MJ, Zhang C, Liang L, et al. Fasting serum glucose, thyroid-stimulating hormone, and thyroid hormones and risk of papillary thyroid cancer: a case-control study. Head Neck. 2019;41:2277–84.
30. Kuijpens JL, Nyklíctek I, Louwman MW, Weetman TA, Pop VJ, Coebergh JW. Hypothyroidism might be related to breast cancer in post-menopausal women. Thyroid. 2005;15:1253–9.
31. Brandt J, Borgquist S, Manjer J. Prospectively measured thyroid hormones and thyroid peroxidase antibodies in relation to risk of different breast cancer subgroups: a Malmö Diet and Cancer Study. Cancer Causes Control. 2015;26:1093–104.
32. Tosovic A, Becker C, Bondeson AG, et al. Prospectively measured thyroid hormones and thyroid peroxidase antibodies in relation to breast cancer risk. Int J Cancer. 2012;131:2126–33.
33. Kim EY, Chang Y, Lee KH, et al. Serum concentration of thyroid hormones in abnormal and euthyroid ranges and breast cancer risk: a cohort study. Int J Cancer. 2019;145:3257–66.
34. Ortega-Olvera C, Ulloa-Aguirre A, Ángeles-Llerenas A, et al. Thyroid hormones and breast cancer association according to menopausal status and body mass index. Breast Cancer Res. 2018;20:94.
35. Chan YX, Knuiman MW, Divitini ML, Brown SJ, Walsh J, Yeap BB. Lower TSH and higher free thyroxine predict incidence of prostate but not breast, colorectal or lung cancer. Eur J Endocrinol. 2017;177:297–308.
36. Shi XZ, Jin X, Xu P, Shen HM. Relationship between breast cancer and levels of serum thyroid hormones and antibodies: a meta-analysis. Asian Pac J Cancer Prev. 2014;15:6643–7.
37. Jiskra J, Límanová Z, Barkmanová J, Smutek D, Friedmannová Z. Autoimmune thyroid diseases in women with breast cancer and colorectal cancer. Physiol Res. 2004;53:693–702.
38. Wu CC, Yu YY, Yang HC, et al. Levothyroxine use and the risk of breast cancer: a nation-wide population-based case-control study. Arch Gynecol Obstet. 2018;298:389–96.
39. Mondul AM, Weinstein SJ, Bosworth T, Remaley AT, Virtamo J, Albanes D. Circulating thyroxine, thyroid-stimulating hormone, and hypothyroid status and the risk of prostate cancer. PLoS One. 2012;7:e47730.
40. Puhr HC, Wolf P, Berghoff AS, Schoppmann SF, Preusser M, Ilhan-Mutlu A. Elevated free thyroxine levels are associated with poorer overall survival in patients with gastroesophageal cancer: a retrospective single center analysis. Horm Cancer. 2020;11:42–51.
41. Boursi B, Haynes K, Mamtani R, Yang YX. Thyroid dysfunction, thyroid hormone replacement and colorectal cancer risk. J Natl Cancer Inst. 2015;107:djv084.
42. Pinter M, Haupt L, Hucke F, et al. The impact of thyroid hormones on patients with hepatocellular carcinoma. PLoS One. 2017;12:e0181878.
43. Sarosiek K, Gandhi AV, Saxena S, et al. Hypothyroidism in pancreatic cancer: role of exogenous thyroid hormone in tumor invasion-preliminary observations. J Thyroid Res. 2016;2016:2454989.

44. Uzair ID, Conte Grand J, Flamini MI, Sanchez AM. Molecular actions of thyroid hormone on breast cancer cell migration and invasion via cortactin/N-WASP. Front Endocrinol (Lausanne). 2019;10:139.
45. Hsieh MT, Wang LM, Changou CA, et al. Crosstalk between integrin αvβ3 and ERα contributes to thyroid hormone-induced proliferation of ovarian cancer cells. Oncotarget. 2017;8(15):24237–49.
46. Shinderman-Maman E, Cohen K, Weingarten C, et al. The thyroid hormone-αvβ3 integrin axis in ovarian cancer: regulation of gene transcription and MAPK-dependent proliferation. Oncogene. 2016;35:1977–87.
47. Davis PJ, Mousa SA, Schechter GP, Lin HY. Platelet ATP, thyroid hormone receptor on integrin αvβ3 and cancer metastasis. Horm Cancer. 2020;11:13–6.
48. Weingarten C, Jenudi Y, Tshuva RY, et al. The interplay between epithelial-mesenchymal transition (EMT) and the thyroid hormones-αvβ3 axis in ovarian cancer. Horm Cancer. 2018;9:22–32.
49. Schmohl KA, Mueller AM, Dohmann M, et al. Integrin αvβ3-mediated effects of thyroid hormones on mesenchymal stem cells in tumor angiogenesis. Thyroid. 2019;29:1843–57.
50. Chin YT, Wei PL, Ho Y, et al. Thyroxine inhibits resveratrol-caused apoptosis by PD-L1 in ovarian cancer cells. Endocr Relat Cancer. 2018;25:533–45.
51. Lin HY, Chin YT, Yang YC, et al. Thyroid hormone, cancer, and apoptosis. Compr Physiol. 2016;6:1221–37.
52. Meng R, Tang HY, Westfall J, et al. Crosstalk between integrin αvβ3 and estrogen receptor-α is involved in thyroid hormone-induced proliferation in human lung carcinoma cells. PLoS One. 2011;6:e27547.
53. Cicatiello AG, Ambrosio R, Dentice M. Thyroid hormone promotes differentiation of colon cancer stem cells. Mol Cell Endocrinol. 2017;459:84–9.
54. Catalano V, Dentice M, Ambrosio R, et al. Activated thyroid hormone promotes differentiation and chemotherapeutic sensitization of colorectal cancer stem cells by regulating Wnt and BMP4 signaling. Cancer Res. 2016;76:1237–44.
55. Wang T, Xia L, Ma S, et al. Hepatocellular carcinoma: thyroid hormone promotes tumorigenicity through inducing cancer stem-like cell self-renewal. Sci Rep. 2016;6:25183.
56. Kotolloshi R, Mirzakhani K, Ahlburg J, Kraft F, Pungsrinont T, Baniahmad A. Thyroid hormone induces cellular senescence in prostate cancer cells through induction of DEC1. J Steroid Biochem Mol Biol. 2020;201:105689.
57. Heublein S, Mayr D, Meindl A, et al. Thyroid hormone receptors predict prognosis in BRCA1 associated breast cancer in opposing ways. PLoS One. 2015;10:e0127072.
58. Jerzak KJ, Cockburn J, Pond GR, et al. Thyroid hormone receptor α in breast cancer: prognostic and therapeutic implications. Breast Cancer Res Treat. 2015;149:293–301.
59. Ditsch N, Toth B, Himsl I, et al. Thyroid hormone receptor (TR)alpha and TRbeta expression in breast cancer. Histol Histopathol. 2013;28:227–37.
60. Kim WG, Zhu X, Kim DW, Zhang L, Kebebew E, Cheng SY. Reactivation of the silenced thyroid hormone receptor β gene expression delays thyroid tumor progression. Endocrinology. 2013;154:25–35.
61. Bolf EL, Gillis NE, Barnum MS, et al. The thyroid hormone receptor-RUNX2 Axis: a novel tumor suppressive pathway in breast cancer. Horm Cancer. 2020;11:34–41.
62. Carr FE, Tai PW, Barnum MS, et al. Thyroid hormone receptor-β (TRβ) mediates runt-related transcription factor 2 (Runx2) expression in thyroid cancer cells: a novel signaling pathway in thyroid cancer. Endocrinology. 2016;157:3278–92.
63. Shao W, Kuhn C, Mayr D, et al. Cytoplasmic and nuclear forms of thyroid hormone receptor β1 are inversely associated with survival in primary breast cancer. Int J Mol Sci. 2020;21:330.
64. Kowalik MA, Puliga E, Cabras L, et al. Thyroid hormone inhibits hepatocellular carcinoma progression via induction of differentiation and metabolic reprogramming. J Hepatol. 2020;72:1159–69.

65. Wu SM, Cheng WL, Liao CJ, et al. Negative modulation of the epigenetic regulator, UHRF1, by thyroid hormone receptors suppresses liver cancer cell growth. Int J Cancer. 2015;137:37–49.
66. Wojcicka A, Piekielko-Witkowska A, Kedzierska H, et al. Epigenetic regulation of thyroid hormone receptor beta in renal cancer. PLoS One. 2014;9:e97624.
67. Ichijo S, Furuya F, Shimura H, et al. Activation of the RhoB signaling pathway by thyroid hormone receptor β in thyroid cancer cells. PLoS One. 2014;9:e116252.
68. Davis PJ, Lin HY, Hercbergs AA, Keating KA, Mousa SA. How thyroid hormone works depends upon cell type, receptor type, and hormone analogue: implications in cancer growth. Discov Med. 2019;27:111–7.
69. Mousa SA, Glinsky GV, Lin HY, et al. Contributions of thyroid hormone to cancer metastasis. Biomedicine. 2018;6:89.
70. Krashin E, Piekielko-Witkowska A, Ellis M, Ashur-Fabian O. Thyroid hormones and cancer: a comprehensive review of preclinical and clinical studies. Front Endocrinol (Lausanne). 2019;10:59.
71. Gu G, Gelsomino L, Covington KR, et al. Targeting thyroid hormone receptor beta in triple-negative breast cancer. Breast Cancer Res Treat. 2015;150:535–45.
72. Shinderman-Maman E, Cohen K, Moskovich D, et al. Thyroid hormones derivatives reduce proliferation and induce cell death and DNA damage in ovarian cancer. Sci Rep. 2017;7:16475.
73. Leith JT, Mousa SA, Hercbergs A, Lin HY, Davis PJ. Radioresistance of cancer cells, integrin αvβ3 and thyroid hormone. Oncotarget. 2018;9:37069–75.
74. Goemann IM, Marczyk VR, Romitti M, Wajner SM, Maia AL. Current concepts and challenges to unravel the role of iodothyronine deiodinases in human neoplasias. Endocr Relat Cancer. 2018;25:R625–45.
75. Casula S, Bianco AC. Thyroid hormone deiodinases and cancer. Front Endocrinol (Lausanne). 2012;3:74.

Practical Application of Levothyroxine-Based Therapy

Takashi Akamizu

Levothyroxine (LT4) is a natural, endogenous hormone. Adverse events associated with this treatment are mostly symptoms of over-treatment (a state of functional thyrotoxicosis), which can be avoided by careful titration of the LT4 dosage to keep thyrotropin within an appropriate reference range that is relevant to the needs of the individual patient.

1 Introduction

The intention of this chapter is to complete this book on the role of levothyroxine (LT4) in the management of thyroid dysfunction, with a summary of the practical application of this treatment. The focus of the chapter will be on the management of hypothyroidism; for information relating to the implications of TSH-suppressive doses of LT4, the reader should consult chapter "Levothyroxine and Bone" and chapter "Levothyroxine and Cancer". I will consider how to dose LT4, how patients should take it and the tolerability and safety implications long-term LT4-based therapy. This approach will involve reviewing important information from prescribing documentation for preparations of LT4 from Europe [1] and the USA [2], as these impact on clinical practice across a large area of the world beyond the borders of those regions. For example, physicians in Middle-Eastern countries are influenced by, but not bound by, labelling from both of these regions. Physicians should always consult their local labelling, where available, before prescribing LT4, however. Finally, the chapter will provide a resource of guidelines for the management of hypothyroidism around the world.

T. Akamizu (✉)
Wakayama Medical University, Wakayama, Japan

Kuma Hospital, Kobe, Japan
e-mail: akamizu@wakayama-med.ac.jp, akamizu@kuhp.kyoto-u.ac.jp

© The Author(s) 2021
G. J. Kahaly (ed.), *70 Years of Levothyroxine*,
https://doi.org/10.1007/978-3-030-63277-9_10

2 Safety and Tolerability of Levothyroxine

2.1 Avoiding Symptoms of Thyroid Dysfunction

The prescribing documentation for levothyroxine (LT4) products for use in patients with hypothyroidism notes that the adverse events associated with this treatment generally refer to over-treatment with LT4, which induces a state of thyrotoxicosis. Alternatively, inadequate correction of TSH leaves the hypothyroid patient at risk of a range of adverse outcomes, including major adverse cardiovascular events and premature death (see chapter "Levothyroxine and the Heart" for more details) [3, 4]. Accordingly, both over-treatment and under-treatment with LT4 leave the patient with hypothyroidism at increased risk of adverse long-term clinical outcomes, as well as troublesome symptoms of thyroid dysfunction (summarised in Fig. 1).

- Weight loss[a,b]
- Fatigue[a,b]
- Heat intolerance[b]
- Cardiac arrhythmias (e.g. atrial fibrillation, extrasystoles) and palpitations[a,b]
- Tachycardia[a,b]
- Increased blood pressure[b]
- Diarrhoea[a,b]
- Angina[a], myocardial infarction/ cardiac arrest[b]
- Cephalalgia[a]
- Muscle weakness, cramps or spasm[a,b]
- Flushing, rash[a,b]
- Hair loss[b]
- Fever[a,b]
- Vomiting[a,b]

- Weight gain
- Fatigue
- Sensitivity to cold
- Constipation
- Depression
- Slow movements and thoughts
- Muscle aches and weakness
- Muscle cramps
- Dry/scaly skin
- Brittle hair and nails
- Loss of libido
- Carpal tunnel syndrome
- Irregular or heavy menstruation

- Pseudotumor cerebri[a]
- Tremor[a,b]
- Disordered menstruation/infertility[a,b]
- Increased appetite[b]
- Restlessness[a]/hyperactivity[b]
- Insomnia[a,b]
- Headache[b]
- Dyspnoea[b]
- Nervousness/anxiety/irritability/emotional instability[b]
- Excessive sweating (hyperhidrosis)[a,b]
- Abnormal liver function tests[b]
- Decreased bone mineral density[b]

Symptoms similar to hypothyroidism
(LT4 dosage too low)

Symptoms of thyrotoxicosis
(LT4 dosage too high)

Fig. 1 Overview of symptoms arising from suboptimal dosing of levothyroxine in patients with hypothyroidism. Symptoms of hyperthyroidism/thyrotoxicosis were from [a]the European Summary of Product Characteristics [1] and [b]US Prescribing Information [2] for levothyroxine (LT4) products. Symptoms of hypothyroidism were as listed by the United Kingdom National Health Service [3]

The goal of LT4 management is thus to optimise the LT4 dosage [1–5]. It is important to note that symptoms of thyroid dysfunction are often non-specific in nature, and in some cases similar symptoms are identified for both under- and over-treatment with LT4.

Increased actions of catecholamines are a feature of thyrotoxicosis, including following an overdose of LT4 [6]. Accordingly, a number of adverse consequences of thyrotoxicosis following over-treatment with LT4 are mediated via over-stimulation of β-adrenoceptors, such as tachycardia, anxiety, agitation and hyperkinesia. Treatment with a β-blocker may be helpful here. The European prescribing documentation also warns that over dosage of LT4 may increase the risk of acute psychosis (especially in patients at risk of this condition), and that long-term abuse of LT4 has been associated with cardiovascular death. Seizures are another rare complication of LT4 therapy [2].

The possibility of increased risk of cardiovascular events (see chapter "Levothyroxine and the Heart"), or of osteoporotic fractures (see chapter "Levothyroxine and Bone"), are among the more serious long-term consequences of thyrotoxicosis. This is a particular concern where TSH-suppressive doses of LT4 are administered. Long-term treatment with high doses of LT4 may be administered after total thyroidectomy for well-differentiated thyroid carcinoma in order to suppress secretion of TSH from the pituitary (e.g. see chapter "Levothyroxine and Cancer"), which induces a thyrotoxic status similar to a chronic form of subclinical hyperthyroidism [7–9]. These patients are likely to be at elevated risk of long-term adverse effects, such as those in the cardiovascular system (possible increased risk of adverse cardiovascular events, see chapter "Levothyroxine and the Heart") or the skeleton (possible increased risk of osteoporosis and fractures, especially in those at increased risk, such as postmenopausal women—see chapter "Levothyroxine and Bone").

2.2 Adverse Reactions to the LT4 Tablet Itself

Additionally, as with any medicinal product, hypersensitivity reactions in the skin or respiratory system may occur rarely in response to components of the LT4 tablet, possibly including LT4 itself [1, 2]. Such reactions tend to manifest with symptoms, such as urticaria, eczema-like rashes, fever and disturbances of liver function tests, and may persist when different LT4 products are prescribed [10–13]. Excipients vary somewhat between LT4 preparations, and so changes the brand of LT4 may help to resolve the issue; however, hypersensitivity to LT4 itself may effectively prevent the effective management of hypothyroidism [14]. Procedures for oral desensitisation have been described, where administration of successively increasing LT4 dosages (e.g. at 30-min intervals, from an initial dose as low as 0.01 µg) enable subsequent chronic therapy with doses of LT4 that are clinically effective [10–13].

3 How to Prescribe and Take Levothyroxine

Hypothyroidism usually requires patients to take LT4 for life. Accordingly, patients must be educated on how to take their LT4 tablets correctly, to have any chance of achieving stable, euthyroid-like thyroid hormone function over the long term (Table 1). Food has a markedly inhibitory effect on the absorption and bioavailability of LT4 (see chapter "Administration and Pharmacokinetics of Levothyroxine"). Accordingly, it is important that LT4 is taken on an empty stomach, and that no

Table 1 How to take levothyroxine (LT4): examples from products available in Europe and in the USA

	Europe	USA
Dosing frequency for the management of hypothyroidism	One tablet, once-daily	One tablet, once-daily
When to take LT4	30 min before breakfast on an empty stomach	30–60 min before breakfast on an empty stomach
Typical starting doses		
Adults with hypothyroidism	25–50 μg[a]	100–125 μg (70 kg adult)[e]
Elderly	12.5 μg[a]	12–25 μg
Adults with hypothyroidism + CHD	12.5 μg	12–25 μg
Infants/neonates with CH[b]	10–15 μg/kg	10–15 μg/kg[b,f]
Children	12.5–50 μg	Varies[f]
Typical dose adjustments	Every 2–4 weeks (elderly: 12.5 mg every 2 weeks)	12.5–25 μg every 4–6 weeks (6–8 weeks for elderly)
Typical maintenance doses		
Adults with hypothyroidism	100–200 μg/day	About 1.6 μg/kg
Adults with hypothyroidism + CHD	As above, possibly lower[c]	May be <1 μg/kg (elderly + CHD)
Children	100–150 μg/m²	Varies[f]
Elderly	As for adults, possibly lower	May be <1 μg/kg
TSH suppression post-surgery for well-differentiated thyroid cancer	150–300 μg	Usually >2 μg/kg

Contraindications to LT4	• Hypersensitivity to LT4 or excipients
	• Untreated:
	
	  – Adrenal insufficiency
	  – Pituitary insufficiency
	  – Thyrotoxicosis
	
	• Acute MI
	• Acute myocarditis
	• Acute pancreatitis
	• Use with anti-thyroid agent during pregnancy
		• Untreated adrenal insufficiency

Table 1 (continued)

	Europe	USA

Special warnings and precautions	• Exclude/treat diseases of:
	
	  – CV system[d]
	  – Pituitary
	  – Adrenals
	
	• TSH autonomy
	• Psychosis
	• Risk of osteoporosis
		• Patients with CHD (especially elderly)
		• Myxoedema coma
		• Acute adrenal crisis (patients with adrenal insufficiency)
		• Worsened glycaemic control
		• Risk of osteoporosis

Compiled from information presented in Refs. [1, 2]

[a]The exact starting dose depends on other factors, such as thyrotropin (TSH) level and body weight

[b]For the first 3 months of life

[c]Start low, go slow in adults with hypothyroidism and CHD, and consider the possibility of a lower maintenance dose than in an adult without CHD

[d]Angina, arteriosclerosis, hypertension

[e]Healthy, non-elderly patients with recent onset hypothyroidism

[f]Guidance on doses for children of different ages is provided

food, coffee, etc. is consumed for at least 30 min (according to European guidance, and up to 1 h, according to guidance from the USA) after taking the LT4 tablet (half a glass of water or so is permitted to allow the tablet to be taken). The usual recommendation is to take LT4 first thing in the morning, so that the 30 min before needing to eat is occupied by the usual morning rituals of bathing, etc. In principle, LT4 can be taken at bedtime although the need to wait for 3 h after the evening meal before taking the tablet [15, 16] may be difficult to maintain consistently, with a consequent reduction in the stability of LT4's biological actions.

The administration of LT4 in the management of hypothyroidism is tailored to the individual needs of the patient, according to an individually determined target for thyrotropin (thyroid-stimulating hormone, TSH) [17, 18]. Starting and maintenance doses (Table 1) vary according to a number of factors, including the therapeutic indication for LT4, age and comorbidity (especially where there is concomitant cardiovascular disease). Starting doses of LT4 for the management of hypothyroidism, and perhaps long-term targets for the TSH level, are likely to be lower in patients with certain comorbidities. US labelling for LT4 permits initiating treatment at the estimated full LT4 dose for T4 replacement in a patient with recent onset hypothyroidism uncomplicated by comorbidities, however. The speed at which the LT4 dose is titrated to achieve control of TSH also varies with the characteristics of the individual patient.

Contraindications and warnings associated with LT4 usually relate to use in patients with comorbidities where the potential harm of accidental over-treatment with LT4 is highest. These relate especially to comorbidities in the cardiovascular and adrenal systems and the risk of osteoporosis (Table 1).

4 Overview of Guidelines on the Management of Hypothyroidism

This book has drawn on major guidelines from Europe and the USA to summarise the current role of LT4 in the management of hypothyroidism, as described in its individual chapters. Many other sources of guidance are available; however, we have listed some of these in Table 2, alongside those from Europe and the USA, as a resource our readers in these areas [17–32]. For clarity and brevity, we have restricted this slit to guidelines that impact on the management of hypothyroidism: please consult chapter "Levothyroxine and Cancer" for detailed information on the use of LT4 in the management of differentiated thyroid cancer.

Table 2 Selection of guidelines for the management of hypothyroidism

Ref.	Country/region	Sponsor	Year	Scope
[20]	International	Expert panel	2019	• Thyroid hormone treatment for subclinical hypothyroidism
[21]	International	ES	2012	• Management of thyroid dysfunction in pregnancy and post-partum
[22]	Europe	ETA	2014	• Subclinical hypothyroidism in pregnancy and in children
[17]	Europe	ETA	2013	• Subclinical hypothyroidism, in younger (<65 years) and elderly patients
[18]	USA	ATA	2017	• Thyroid disease in pregnancy and post-partum • Includes content on iodine deficiency, and management of overt and subclinical hypothyroidism
[19]	USA	ATA	2014	• Broad in scope: Includes hypothyroidism associated with iodine deficiency, and management of congenital, overt and subclinical hypothyroidism • Includes special populations (paediatric subjects, elderly, pregnancy, patients who are non-adherent to LT4)
[23]	USA	AACE/ATA	2012	• Broad scope covering multiple aspects of hypothyroidism
[24]	Latin America	LATS	2013	• Includes hypothyroidism associated with iodine deficiency, and management of overt and subclinical hypothyroidism • Includes special populations (elderly, pregnancy)
[25]	Japan	JTA	NA	• Diagnosis of hypothyroidism (and other aspects of thyroid dysfunction)
[26]	UK	NICE	2019	• Thyroid dysfunction, including primary hypothyroidism, subclinical hypothyroidism, hyperthyroidism, thyroid enlargement
[27]	UK	BTA	2016	• Management of primary and overt hypothyroidism
[28]	UK	BTA	2007	• Use of thyroid extract and LT4 + LT3 combinations
[29]	UK	ACB, BTA, BTF	2006	• Use of thyroid function tests

Table 2 (continued)

Ref.	Country/region	Sponsor	Year	Scope
[30]	Canada (Alberta)	TOP	2014	• Concise, at-a-glance summary of management options for primary hypothyroidism
[31]	Australia	DoH	2019	• Management of hypothyroidism during pregnancy
[32]	Australia, New Zealand	RCGPA	2019	• Thyroid function testing in adults

Guidelines published in or after 2010 are considered here. *AACE* American Association of Clinical Endocrinologists, *ACB* Association for Clinical Biochemistry, *ATA* American Thyroid Association, *BTA* British Thyroid Association, *BTF* British Thyroid Foundation, *DoH* Department of Health, *ES* Endocrine Society, *ETA* European Thyroid Association, *JTA* Japan Thyroid Association, *LATS* Latin American Thyroid Association, *NA* not available from source, *RCPA* Royal College of Pathologists of Australia, *TOP* towards optimised practice, *LT4* levothyroxine

Guidelines from the American Thyroid Association tend to be comprehensive and cover multiple aspects of thyroid dysfunction, while those from the European Thyroid Association tend to focus on specific aspects, such as subclinical hypothyroidism in special patient populations. Hypothyroidism is especially difficult to manage in the setting of pregnancy and breastfeeding, and guidelines from these expert societies address this need. Regional guidelines are available from Latin America, also, as well as individual countries including the UK and Japan.

5 Conclusions

The LT4 molecule is identical chemically with the endogenous thyroid hormone, T4. Accordingly, other than rare hypersensitivity reactions to excipients or other pharmaceutical components of the LT4 tablet, symptoms reported by people with hypothyroidism receiving LT4 treatment will relate to the dosage of LT4 they receive, and the severity of their thyroid dysfunction. Novel, re-engineered formulations of LT4 have the potential to increase the reproducibility and constancy of exposure to LT4 during long-term management, which may help to achieve optimal dose titration of LT4 (see chapter "Administration and Pharmacokinetics of Levothyroxine" for an example). Some patients are given supra-physiologic doses of LT4 as a deliberate part of their management, such as those undergoing LT4-based suppression of TSH levels to reduce the risk of disease recurrence after thyroidectomy for thyroid cancer, or to reduce the growth and potential for malignancy of thyroid nodules. Research is continuing to determine the most appropriate LT4-based management algorithms for these patients, to optimise their long-term clinical outcomes.

We, the authors, hope that you have enjoyed reading this book, and that you have found it useful in your clinical practice.

References

1. Merck KgAA. Euthyrox®. Summary of product characteristics.
2. US Prescribing Information for Synthroid®, a trademark of AbbieVie Inc. Available at www. synthroid.com. Accessed Jul 2020.
3. Thayakaran R, Adderley NJ, Sainsbury C, et al. Thyroid replacement therapy, thyroid stimulating hormone concentrations, and long term health outcomes in patients with hypothyroidism: longitudinal study. BMJ. 2019;l4892:366.
4. Lillevang-Johansen M, Abrahamsen B, Jørgensen HL, Brix TH, Hegedüs L. Over- and under-treatment of hypothyroidism is associated with excess mortality: a register-based cohort study. Thyroid. 2018;28:566–74.
5. National Health Service. Symptoms—underactive thyroid (hypothyroidism). Available at https://www.nhs.uk/conditions/underactive-thyroid-hypothyroidism/symptoms/. Accessed May 2020.
6. Silva JE, Bianco SD. Thyroid-adrenergic interactions: physiological and clinical implications. Thyroid. 2008;18:157–65.
7. Biondi B, Filetti S, Schlumberger M. Thyroid-hormone therapy and thyroid cancer: a reassessment. Nat Clin Pract Endocrinol Metab. 2005;1:32–40.
8. Biondi B, Cooper DS. Benefits of thyrotropin suppression versus the risks of adverse effects in differentiated thyroid cancer. Thyroid. 2010;20:135–46.
9. Heemstra KA, Hamdy NA, Romijn JA, Smit JW. The effects of thyrotropin-suppressive therapy on bone metabolism in patients with well-differentiated thyroid carcinoma. Thyroid. 2006;16:583–91.
10. Dortas SD, De Araujo FM, Souza CR, et al. Drug rash induced by levothyroxine and oral desensitization. World Allergy Organ J. 2015;8:A21. Available at https://waojournal.biomed-central.com/articles/10.1186/1939-4551-8-S1-A21. Accessed Jul 2020.
11. Fevzi D, Mustafa G, Ozgur K, et al. Successful oral desensitization to levothyroxine. Ann Allergy Asthma Immunol. 2013;111:146–7.
12. Guzmán MA, Sepúlveda C, Liberman C, et al. Desensibilización a levotiroxina. Caso clínico [Successful oral desensitization to levothyroxine. Report of one case]. Rev Med Chil. 2018;146:394–8.
13. Sala A, Labrador-Horrillo M, Guilarte M, Luengo O, Rueda M. Immediate-type hypersensitivity reaction to levothyroxine and desensitization. Ann Allergy Asthma Immunol 100. 5:P513–4.
14. Siddiqui MS, Shotliff K. Levothyroxine—not all tablets are the same. Prescriber 15 Jul 2019. Available at https://www.prescriber.co.uk/article/levothyroxine-not-all-tablets-are-the-same. Accessed Jul 2020.
15. Benvenga S, Bartolone L, Squadrito S, Lo Giudice F, Trimarchi F. Delayed intestinal absorption of levothyroxine. Thyroid. 1995;5:249–53.
16. Wenzel KW, Kirschsieper HE. Aspects of the absorption of oral L-thyroxine in normal man. Metabolism. 1977;26:1–8.
17. Pearce SH, Brabant G, Duntas LH, et al. ETA guideline: management of subclinical hypothyroidism. Eur Thyroid J. 2013;2:215–28.
18. Alexander EK, Pearce EN, Brent GA, et al. Guidelines of the American Thyroid Association for the diagnosis and management of thyroid disease during pregnancy and the postpartum. Thyroid. 2017;27:315–89.
19. Jonklaas J, Bianco AC, Bauer AJ, et al. Guidelines for the treatment of hypothyroidism: prepared by the American Thyroid Association Task Force on Thyroid Hormone Replacement. Thyroid. 2014;24:1670–751.
20. Bekkering GE, Agoritsas T, Lytvyn L, et al. Thyroid hormones treatment for subclinical hypothyroidism: a clinical practice guideline. BMJ. 2019;l2006:365.
21. De Groot L, Abalovich M, Alexander EK, et al. Management of thyroid dysfunction during pregnancy and postpartum: an Endocrine Society clinical practice guideline. J Clin Endocrinol Metab. 2012;97:2543–65.

22. Lazarus J, Brown RS, Daumerie C, Hubalewska-Dydejczyk A, Negro R, Vaidya B. 2014 European Thyroid Association guidelines for the management of subclinical hypothyroidism in pregnancy and in children. Eur Thyroid J. 2014;3:76–94.
23. Garber JR, Cobin RH, Gharib H, et al. Clinical practice guidelines for hypothyroidism in adults: cosponsored by the American Association of Clinical Endocrinologists and the American Thyroid Association. Thyroid. 2012;22:1200–35.
24. Brenta G, Vaisman M, Sgarbi JA, et al. Clinical practice guidelines for the management of hypothyroidism. Arq Bras Endocrinol Metabol. 2013;57:265–91.
25. Japan Thyroid Association. Guidelines. Available at http://www.japanthyroid.jp/en/guidelines. html. Accessed Jul 2020.
26. Thyroid disease: assessment and management. NICE guideline [NG145]. Nov 2019. Available at https://www.nice.org.uk/guidance/ng145/chapter/Recommendations. Accessed Jul 2020.
27. Okosieme O, Gilbert J, Abraham P, et al. Management of primary hypothyroidism: statement by the British Thyroid Association Executive Committee. Clin Endocrinol (Oxf). 2016;84:799–808.
28. British Thyroid Association Executive Committee. Armour thyroid (USP) and combined thyroxine/tri-iodothyronine as thyroid hormone replacement. Feb 2007. Available at https://www.british-thyroid-association.org/sandbox/bta2016/bta_statement_on_the_use_of_armour_thyroid_and_combined_t4_and_t3.pdf. Accessed Jul 2020.
29. Association for Clinical Biochemistry, British Thyroid Association, British Thyroid Foundation. UK guidelines for the use of thyroid function tests. Available at https://www.british-thyroid-association.org/sandbox/bta2016/uk_guidelines_for_the_use_of_thyroid_function_tests.pdf. Accessed Jul 2020.
30. Toward Optimized Practice (TOP) Endocrine Working Group. Investigation and management of primary thyroid dysfunction. Clinical practice guideline. April 2014. Available at https://actt.albertadoctors.org/CPGs/Lists/CPGDocumentList/thyroid-guideline.pdf. Accessed Jul 2020.
31. Australian Government Department of Health. Pregnancy Care Guidelines. 46 Thyroid dysfunction. Available at https://www.health.gov.au/resources/pregnancy-care-guidelines/part-g-targeted-maternal-health-tests/thyroid-dysfunction. Accessed Jul 2020.
32. Royal College of Pathologists of Australia. Position Statement. Thyroid function testing for adult diagnosis and monitoring. Available at https://www.rcpa.edu.au/Library/College-Policies/Position-Statements/Thyroid-Function-Testing-for-Adult-Diagnosis-and-M. Accessed Jul 2020.

Printed in the United States
by Baker & Taylor Publisher Services